THE GUT HEALING
PROTOCOL

An 8-Week, Holistic Program
for Rebalancing Your Microbiome

Kale Brock

Library of Congress Cataloging-in-Publication Data

Names: Brock, Kale, author.
Title: The gut healing protocol : an 8-week, holistic program for rebalancing
  your microbiome / by Kale Brock.
Description: Third edition. | Oxnard, CA : Primal Blueprint Publishing,
  [2018] | Revised edition of: The gut healing protocol : an 8 week,
  holistic guide to re-balancing your gut. Second edition. [Australia] :
  Kale Brock, 2017. | Includes bibliographical references and index.
Identifiers: LCCN 2017048901 (print) | LCCN 2017049652 (ebook) | ISBN
  9781939563446 (ebook) | ISBN 9781939563439 (paperback)
Subjects: LCSH: Digestive organs--Diseases--Diet therapy--Popular works. |
  Gastrointestinal system--Diseases--Diet therapy--Popular works. | Cooking
  (Natural foods)
Classification: LCC RC806 (ebook) | LCC RC806 .B76 2018 (print) | DDC
  616.3/30654--dc23
LC record available at https://lccn.loc.gov/2017048901

Editor: Tracy Kearns
Cover Design: Janée Meadows
Interior Design and Layout: Caroline De Vita
Photos of Kale by Spencer Frost. Recipe photos by Kenya Addison at Rhythm of Food.
Copyediting, Proofreading, and Indexing: Tim Tate

Primal Blueprint Publishing, 1641 S. Rose Ave., Oxnard, CA 93033
Please contact the publisher with any questions, concerns, and feedback, or to obtain
quantity discounts.
888-774-6259 or 310-317-4414
email: info@primalblueprintpublishing.com, or visit PrimalBlueprintPublishing.com.

Contents

Testimonials

Here's how some have fared while applying the Gut Healing Protocol. These are real-life stories from everyday people like you and me who took charge of their health, applied basic, gut-nourishing principles, and experienced an incredible result.

Dr. Nick Gentile:

*I expected big things from Kale's **Gut Healing Protocol**, yet even still I was surprised and amazed by the results. Not only did I lose 9kgs, improve my energy, fortify my immune system and greatly speed up my recovery from exercise, but most importantly my digestion improved out of sight. I'm now free of the stomach pain and bloating that I experienced on a daily basis and I'm looking forward to maintaining the changes I've put in place long into the future! I can't recommend this program highly enough.*

Taela Old:

I thought I was doing right by my body… I was exercising a lot between work shifts and I thought I was "eating healthy," but I started to gain a lot of weight. I was experiencing terrible pains in my stomach as well as bloating and I was struggling with constant fatigue. I knew I had to change my lifestyle but I had no idea where to start since I couldn't understand what I was doing wrong.

Then a miracle happened! I was introduced to the idea of doing Kale Brock's Gut Healing Protocol. I was initially really scared of the idea, but I decided to give it a shot.

As I discovered, coupling this Gut Healing Protocol with my exercise programs, my whole lifestyle changed dramatically. I noticed in a very short amount of time that my mind was improving as well as my body image! Since finishing the gut cleanse, I have no desire to go back to how I was eating beforehand because I am the healthiest and happiest I have ever been!

Andrea Dillon:

Prior to the program, I was already on a fairly clean diet, but over time had allowed a few habits I had previously eradicated to creep back into my lifestyle. As a result, I was suffering from candidiasis and bloating again and was feeling frustrated. Kale's program required dedication and organization, but it was well worth the effort and gradually my symptoms began to subside. It was so empowering to be making such great food choices for each meal, and knowing that everything you ate was improving your health and allowing your stomach to heal.

There are many more testimonials at:
www.kalebrock.com.au/changedlives.

CHAPTER 1

Introduction

The gut. The gut lining. It's one of the hottest topics in science right now. Scientists the world over are scrupulously investigating the role that our microbiome and subsequent functioning of the intestinal lining play in our health and wellbeing. Let me tell you, they're discovering some amazing things, many of which I will share with you in this book.

This book is the result of nine years of my research as a health journalist and coach into how we as everyday people can better look after ourselves in order to experience life to the fullest. This book is not a scientific journal or investigative report, but rather a simple action plan, with validating references, that you can use to improve your gut health and furthermore to improve your overall health and vitality!

The Gut Healing Protocol is an extra tool for your health maintenance "toolbox." It contains principles that I learned from some of my earliest (and still current) healthcare mentors. I've borrowed ideas and principles from prominent doctors who I've interviewed over the years and incorporated philosophical ideas from health leaders and backed them up with scientific references. I've taken ideas from the pages of the thousands of books and articles I've read on health and wellness, and I've tidied it all up into a pretty little package called the Gut Healing Protocol.

I'm not a doctor. I am a normal person, just like you, who was forced to learn about the wonderful thing I live in called the human body. I believe the most powerful thing about this protocol is its simplicity. This is literally a real-food approach to healing the gut lining and improving one's health. It's the approach I had to take to improve my own health when I was a young person, and it's the approach I still harness now to maintain vitality. When I sat down to write this book, I didn't want to overwhelm anyone. I didn't want to create a manifesto that only the most advanced health researcher or practitioner could understand. I wanted to make this book applicable and friendly to the everyday person. Gone are the days when health and wellbeing was reserved only for those considered "alternative." The fantastic news is that asking questions and taking responsibility for one's health is common practice now.

Unfortunately, we have many individuals involved in the health movement who create a picture of holistic health as being niche and unobtainable for common people and this is one of the biggest downfalls of the health movement as it stands right now; the fact that it is viewed as "too hard" or "too weird." I believe that as an educated person on health and wellness, it is my responsibility to convey the health message in a simple, comprehensive, and enjoyable way to the public. Most importantly, my goal is to inspire readers to take action. That is the mission behind all my work in this industry. One of the greatest pleasures I receive from this job is when a reader or listener tells me that they got their health back in control and are now living their life to the fullest because they felt inspired in some way by my work.

Health and wellness is simply a tool to help you achieve your dreams.

This book is called *The Gut Healing Protocol* because it focuses, primarily, on the health of the intestinal lining. For the nerdy, this means tightening up the junctions of the gut epithelium and shutting down over-active inflammatory mechanisms throughout the body so that you can experience optimal bodily function. This is like resetting the gut or figuratively getting a "gut-chiropractic-adjustment." When we calm the system down, we can allow our health and vitality to thrive.

I will be providing you with a lot of information on the mechanisms of the gut and your digestive system, because when you are well-informed, you can make informed decisions.

The current scientific interest in the *microbiome* is discovering that many of our current ailments including arthritis, psoriasis, Hashimoto's, depression, diabetes, asthma, and even heart disease have some origins in the gut. This is probably because our gut and the functioning of the gut lining has a heavy influence on the inflammatory responses which go on throughout the entire body. Your gut is like the body's central dashboard. It has connections to all the different parts of the body and can send signals to and fro. Those signals can either be health-promoting or disease-promoting, and that is controlled by the functioning of the gut itself. By rebalancing the gut *microbiota*, decreasing inflammation, and restoring integrity to the intestinal lining, we can create a digestive environment that is health-promoting!

Microbiota: The individual microbes which inhabit the body.

Microbiome: The sum total of the microbiota population which inhabit the body.

What's so fantastic about the gut message is that it represents a strong intersection between "alternative" health and conventional medicine. For years these fields have remained very separate from one another, often criticizing and attacking the opposing team from afar. But with the accumulation of science confirming gut-health principles as being core to the development and maintenance of wellbeing, these groups are coming together. One of the greatest benefits of this intersection of ideas is that we as consumers will see huge advancements in how disease is treated, if not prevented. Indeed, there are many conventional doctors, as well as many complimentary practitioners who are still "behind the 8 ball" in terms of gut health, and that is why I encourage you to educate yourself on the basics of gut health to ensure you're always making informed decisions about your wellbeing.

When we break down the sometimes complex and overwhelming scientific research, a common theme arises: *most disease and illness can originate or be exacerbated by an imbalance in the gut microbiome and a lack of intestinal integrity.* In other words, when we have too many "bad bugs" and not enough "good bugs" or bacteria, this opens up the doors to inflammation and a leaky gut which in turn leads to immunological challenges in the body. (Leaky gut is covered in-depth in Chapter 3.)

Understand this fundamental point: the core principles of gut healing address the balance of microbes within your gastrointestinal tract and the health of the intestinal lining. These two factors are always at play when we discuss any sort of gut-related illness.

Now, is the gut the root of *all* disease? I certainly don't think so. Although it is extremely important as a fundamental foundation for optimal health and wellness, it's not the be-all and end-all by any means. **Health and wellbeing is far more than the food you put in your mouth and the exercise you do. It is all encompassing. Your job, your relationships, your happiness—all these factors can cause you to be healthy or unhealthy.**

Any imbalance in these areas can result in a disease-like state in the body, but the key factor is that *it is much easier to balance all the areas of health with adequate functioning of the gut than it is without.*

Optimizing the gut is like laying the foundations for a house. You wouldn't build a house out of sticks and straw, would you? You would use strong lumber or bricks or a mixture of both because you want your house to withstand the normal pressures of the weather, screaming children, and social life!

Until we optimize the functioning of the gut, we can always expect challenges to our health and wellbeing, because it is the gut that feeds the entire body with either health-promoting or disease-promoting information.

The simple protocol that I outline in this book is a back-to-basics real-food approach to restoring gut health. It involves basic, paleo-style recipes which I have created or learned and tweaked to ensure that your body has the best chance to decrease the inflammation in your gut to allow your intestinal lining to heal. The protocol is written for *long-term* as well as *short-term* health, because what I've found is those who approach wellness as a *sprint* rather than a marathon are doomed to fail. Think long-term to experience and benefit from health and wellness for the rest of your life!

Being 80% perfect for the rest of your life is far better than being 100% perfect for 12 weeks.

If this book only serves as a reminder to consider your gut health each time you eat, then it has done its job! You may not need to follow "the protocol" if you're not experiencing health issues and simply want to improve your digestion. Or, you may be someone who is actively looking for a solution to your gut-health challenges and that's great, too! Try not to always think of this book as "the program," but rather treat it as a resource for you to start making your own decisions about your health!

Let go of your emotional attachment to food, and use it as a fuel to get you where you want to go.

The principles behind the Gut Health Protocol (GHP) have been used by practitioners the world over to assist patients in rebalancing their gut biome. Amazing experts such as Dr. David Perlmutter, Dr. Natasha Campbell-McBride, and Dr. Raphael Kellman have all contributed incredible insights to the gut health field. It is upon their work that this book and protocol are based.

Although this book is suggested to be an eight-week program, this is a diet for life if you want it to be. For some, it may take 12-16 weeks on the GHP to reach your health goals; it depends on the individual and their state of health.

I've known some people who felt so good after eating and living this way that they don't want to go back to anything else. What I truly love about the information in this book is that it incorporates the development of healthy habits way beyond just a dietary sense. A holistic and *simple* approach to health is often the best way to win!

If you're someone who has "tried everything" and feel like giving up—don't. I am of the firm belief that a body with disease-like symptoms is a body out of balance. You may have already been on a "real food diet" for the last 10 years and still can't get on top of your health, and that's okay. You may be one of the special individuals who will help pave the way toward a brighter future for all. With scientists focusing more on the gut and microbiome, I am confident that most health ailments will be "fixable" in the near future.

The worst thing that can come out of getting serious about your gut health is that you have better foundations to work with when it comes to healing your body.

Throughout this book, I am going to give you tips on how you can best apply gut-nourishing principles. Understanding that readers are in different situations, I distinguish between a "gut-healing protocol" and a "gut-nourishing diet." The former is a good option for those with gut challenges that may present as bloating, pain, indigestion, irregularity or constipation, autoimmune conditions, and more. The latter is a generalized, flexible approach to maintaining gut health over the long term and not necessarily for those recovering from illness. It is for the average person who hasn't had to think about their gut health before, but who wants to work on it at a friendly pace.

We will lead up to the Gut Healing Protocol with a transition week, and we will transition out of the protocol into the more generalized Gut Nourishing Diet for long-term maintenance of our new-found gut health.

You will see how the cultivation of health is not a sprint, but rather a marathon that brings so many compounding benefits to one's life over time. Think about your dreams, goals, and the most precious parts of your life; how would they be actualized or improved if you had optimum health and wellbeing on your side?

I daresay that almost all aspects of your fabulous life are more enjoyable when you're healthy.

So why?

I'm fond of saying that health doesn't have to be the end goal, but it's a powerful tool to get you wherever you want to go. I think this sentiment, this philosophical standpoint, really puts the whole dietary equation into perspective. We need to absolutely respect and honor our bodies by putting in the smartest, most colorful and beautiful fuel we have access to, but we must also focus on the important things in life. I wonder when we are on our way out of this world and into the next, do we think about the meals we ate? The smoothies we drank? Or do we think about the relationships we had, the family we loved, or the exciting adventures we took? I tend to lean towards the latter and it's for that reason that I say to you, let go.

Let go of your emotional attachment to food, and use it as a fuel to get you where you want to go.

Food can still be enjoyable, delectable, and a great area of life, but it's only one part, and I'll boldly suggest only a small part at that. You, my friend, are so much more than what you eat. But still remember, what you eat has the potential to get you so much more out of life.

So, let's get into it. I congratulate you for committing to this journey and I look forward to sharing it with you.

Kale Brock
August 2017
Sydney, Australia

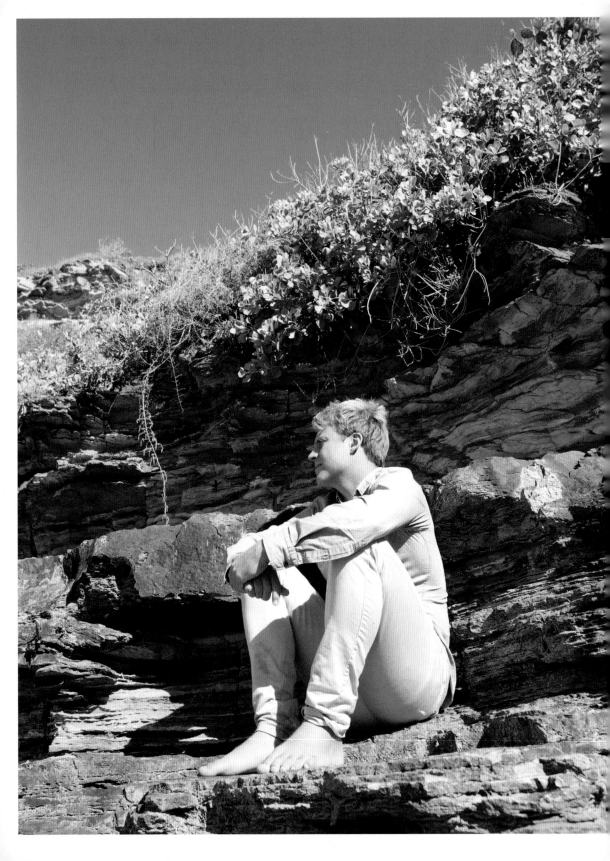

CHAPTER 2

My Story

How did I become a health journalist and coach? It's been a long journey, but I'm going to give you the version I've been sharing with people for the last nine years.

When I was 16, I was diagnosed with Supra-Ventricular-Tachycardia (SVT). I would experience severe arrhythmias to the point where I would almost faint. On the football field. In the car. And in the surf.

One time in particular, I was surfing on a freezing cold morning in South Australia. We were having a blast clambering over marching waves in icy water. As I paddled over one of the crashing waves, my heart felt like it "dropped" out of rhythm. The ensuing tachycardia (abnormal heart beat) was so intense, I could barely paddle. My arms felt like dead weights from the lack of oxygen, and I felt light headed. Deciding the risk of staying in the water wasn't worth it, I managed to tumble to shore with the help of some roaring whitewater.

I felt sick. Weak. Annoyed.

I clambered up to my car and waited for the typical arrhythmia to go away as it normally did after about 3 to 5 minutes. However, this time, it wouldn't go away. I remember because I felt so tired getting into the car. It was incredibly difficult. I just felt like crawling into bed and sleeping, but I still had to work that day, and I needed the money.

I drove 20 minutes down the road to my workplace and sat in the car, closed my eyes, and just prayed to whoever would listen to end this craziness going on in my chest. Why me? All those cliché demands of the universe you make when you're struck down by illness. Fumbling for my phone, I called Mum and told her what was going on. Did I need an ambulance? What should I do? And then it was gone. My heart paused achingly for a moment and seemingly reset its own rhythm. But it was the scariest experience I'd had with my SVT, and it wasn't to be my last, that's for sure.

I visited the cardiologist with Mum soon thereafter, and was sent home with a bunch of battery packs—a portable ECG machine—hooked up to my chest. After 24 hours with the ghastly contraption strapped to my chest (although I did take great pleasure in showing the girls at school), we had nothing to report. All normal, according to the doc.

Further testing was recommended, and a week or so later I found myself grumbling and sweating through a 10-minute jog on a treadmill surrounded by curious doctors staring at me with an expectation that something might happen. The cords that were stuck to my chest whipped and flopped all over the place like a gecko's tail, and the docs seemed unfazed.

Seemingly, nothing eventful was going to take place that day either. But as I slowed down, I felt my heart lift and then drop—the arrhythmia came just in time for the ECG to pick it up. I remember seeing my heart beat rocket on the machine almost into the 200s (bpm).

Delighted murmurs ensued from the men in white coats as they scribbled unintelligible notes on their little clipboards.

"We know what this is Kale. It's SVT."

We were now sitting across from the head cardiologist at Flinders Medical Centre. He was a nice guy. Pretty dry, but relatively friendly. In the weeks following my successful treadmill run, I'd been doing a little research on SVT and what having it would mean. I'd heard that nutrition might help, that I'd be dead by 30, that I'd faint in the ocean and drown… it was all on the table as far as I was concerned.

"What might work is an ablation. This is a minor heart surgery…" *I baulked at this part,* "…where we cut you open, find your heart, and burn away a piece of it."

At that point, he had a little model of the heart in his hands and was taking it apart. All I could imagine at that point were his white gloves, wet and slippery with my blood, tugging at my heart strings (and not in a good way).

Upon asking why he needed to burn something to help me heal, the doc said he was going to burn away the sinoatrial node because it was malfunctioning. He kept saying it *might* fix the problem. Luckily, I knew a family friend at this point who had had that procedure done on several occasions. But he wasn't in the best state of health anymore and was getting weaker and weaker. I didn't want to end up like that.

As the doc continued his intricate exploration of the heart model in front of me, I pondered my future. I needed to keep surfing. That was life. If I couldn't surf… *nothing else mattered.*

It was officially my decision at that point—the ball was in my court, the current in my ventricle, the beat in my atrium… you know what I mean.

"What about nutrition?" I asked.

And that was the defining moment for me. The doc laughed, and in a condescending tone said, "Nutrition's got nothing to do with it."

It was something in the way he waved his hand and looked away that caught my attention, like he knew more than he was letting on. But perhaps he truly didn't believe nutrition was worth considering.

How many of you have experienced something like this? Or know someone who has? I've met thousands of people with similar stories. And unfortunately, this is the sad state of the medical system today—we rarely address the underlying causes of disease, yet it's a critical thing to do.

I do want to point out that I think western medicine is absolutely necessary. Lord forbid if I were ever involved in a car crash and needed surgery, I'd want western medicine. As a friend of mine used to say, you wouldn't want someone out there throwing herbs on you. I'm grateful for the amazing feats achieved by western medicine, but when it comes to disease, we have completely gone down the wrong path, and only now are we slowly realizing this.

And so, I looked at the doctor and considered his very frank dismissal of my idea that nutrition *might* be linked to my condition. There is something reflexive and unintellectual about such a callous dismissal that won't even consider other options. In spite of all its achievements, western medicine too often falls into such habitual thinking.

Aristotle said *it is the mark of an educated mind to entertain a thought without accepting it.*

In that moment, I decided that I was the one who needed to become informed about my condition. I needed to take charge because only I had my best interests at heart and only I could be objective about my approach to recovery. After all I had nothing to lose. I had no reputation at stake, nor was I beholden to any certain treatment. It was time to research my options.

For the following few weeks I researched as much as I could. I even wrote a paper on my condition at school to really have it all sink in. The teacher wrote in the margin, *maybe a future in journalism?* Funny story about that. I learned about blood-sugar levels and how they could potentially affect heart rate. I learned a little about stress and minerals. But my real inflection point, that moment where I struck a decision about my chosen route of recovery, was yet to come.

One evening, I was introduced to an amazing woman, a naturopath, who has now been my mentor over the last 9 years. She was able to teach me in a few short hours, and again over the course of a few months and years, how to rebalance my body, and find my health again. I would need to eat whole foods to supplement the missing nutrients of my diet, and live *holistically*. I *learned* these things very quickly, but I didn't apply all of them for quite a long time. Rather, I began slowly implementing change into my lifestyle at a pace I was comfortable with. The momentum grew and propelled me into a new state of mind until I was excited about health and wellness and could easily say "no" to foods I had previously found addictive.

The first 2 weeks were the hardest, but of course the first 2 weeks of any significant change are *always* the hardest. But I got there and so can you!

The SVT? It turned around in about 6 months! I'm still not 100% improved, but I am definitely 99% better than I was. What really surprised me is that others who have experienced SVT have also benefited from this approach! I have now worked with numerous individuals who have been able to turn around their SVT using simple, holistic principles! I still don't know what it was *exactly* that we did to turn things around, as SVT seems to be a complicated condition with a genetic component. But I do know that it worked, whatever it was!

Currently the health status of most people around the world is quite poor, *especially the Y generation*. We've been brought up on nutrient-depleted food for the most part and have been challenged with accusations of being "lazy" and unmotivated. After you read this book, you might understand why this may be the situation; how is someone supposed to feel excited and enthusiastic when they feel like they have no energy?

Luckily, things are changing, and more than ever we are seeing the youth of the world educating older generations on health and wellness principles. It's been a long journey for some in my family, going from knowing little about health to being very well-informed. But the best part of it is, everybody has enjoyed the journey and is grateful for it. There have been times we've been tested when champagne or beer or chocolate got in the way, but our overall attitude toward food has drastically improved to the point where we can all sit down regularly to a big, gut-friendly meal.

Addressing the health principles I outline in this book saved my life, and I've been lucky enough to share them with others. You can check the stories from some of those who have benefited at kalebrock.com.au/changedlives.

A large part of working with clients in my days as a holistic lifestyle and exercise coach has shown me that now more than ever people are in need of better digestion and gut health! So, I'm very lucky to be sharing with you the culmination of my research into the gut and how to heal it.

CHAPTER 3

Why the GHP?
Gut Science and
the Gut Healing Protocol

This is the big question. Why do I need to consider my gut health? Why would I need to heal my gut lining? Well, if you're currently experiencing any health issues, such as arthritis, thyroid problems, obesity, diabetes, digestive complaints, or fatigue (just to name a few), chances are your gut is not as healthy as it should be. How can such a broad, sweeping statement be made? It can be made on the basis of the thousands of scientific articles coming out on the microbiome and its effects on the human body. The microbiome is simply the group of different bacteria, yeast, parasites and protozoa which live on and inside of you in a symbiotic relationship as integral to the human body as food.

Throughout this book we may use the term "bacteria" as a generalized word for all species of the microbiome, however be sure to recognize that the microbiome is more than just bacteria.

Did you know that the microbial cells in your body can actually outnumber your own cells by up to 10 to 1! You may have heard this statistic before, and it has actually been updated in recent years to show that this ratio varies for individuals. Keep in mind that from a DNA standpoint, microbes outnumber us by 99 to 1! That means that the genetic material in your body is 99% microbial—how interesting is that!

One gram of your poop contains more microbes than there are people on earth—so don't underestimate their relevance.

According to experts, there are 4 main functions of the microbiome.

1. The microbiome manages inflammation and your immune system.

2. The microbiome plays a large role in maintaining the intestinal lining.

3. The microbiome manufactures important chemicals for the entire body, including the brain.

4. The microbiome helps digest and assimilate your food.

Any green thumbs in the audience? Your garden is a great example of an ecosystem dependent on the actions of microbes. Think about the soil in your veggie patch—it is probably the most important factor when it comes to growing healthy plants, right? That's because there are trillions of microbes within that soil that help the plant uptake nutrients. These microbes are *essential* in the health of the plant, and that is why we throw horse manure and compost (*full* of microbes) over our garden plots! Would you try to grow some lettuce or parsley in dried-out, chemically damaged soil?

I produced a TV story on an organic avocado farm. The head farmer shared his philosophy with me.

"We feed the soil to feed the plant; we don't feed the plant itself."

Now substitute the human experience in this sentiment.

"We feed the gut to feed the human; we don't feed the human itself."

Would you try to grow health and vitality from a dried-out, chemically damaged gut/microbiome? You'd have a hard time of it.

When you have disturbances in the gut, you can expect disturbances in a subsequent part of the body! The gut is an integral organ and provides much more to the human experience than just digestion! Science and even mainstream media have now revealed that the balance of microbes in your gut directly influences your health to the point of determining whether you may be at risk for getting illnesses like asthma, diabetes, autism, arthritis, depression, obesity, and allergies.

Professor Charles Mackay, medical researcher at Sydney University says, *"When you look at almost any condition that exists now that didn't exist 40 or 50 years ago, or was much less common 40 or 50 years ago, there is a good chance that it is relating to the actions of the gut microbiota."*[1]

This sentiment is actually not a new one, with healers as far back as Hippocrates putting forward the notion that *all disease begins in the gut.*

Antibiotics and The Post Antibiotic Era

The approach we've taken to health over the past 100 years has certainly included many contradictions to the father of modern medicine's philosophy. Antibiotics have been overprescribed, wreaking havoc on our gastrointestinal health as well as developing resistance to medications from the very bugs we're trying to kill![2]

Throughout high school, I would encounter serious chest infections for up to 3 months at a time, and I would finally take the antibiotics the doctor prescribed only to have them not work! It was only later that I learned that antibiotics are useless when fighting off a viral infection. I also found out that antibiotics act like an atomic bomb in the digestive tract, wiping out the good, bad, and the ugly microbes, often with the latter growing back first!

In fact, a study performed by the Stanford University School of Medicine found "In the first 24 hours after administration of oral antibiotics, a spike in carbohydrate availability takes place in the gut… This transient nutrient surplus, combined with the reduction of friendly gut-dwelling bacteria due to antibiotics, permits at least two potentially deadly pathogens to get a toehold in that otherwise more forbidding environment [C.difficile and Salmonella]."[3]

Antibiotics are also being linked with the development of diabetes now. This is probably due to the fact that the composition of your microbiome has a large influence on your insulin sensitivity. A study carried out in Denmark and published in *The Journal of Clinical Endocrinology and Metabolism* examined 5.6 million people over a 12-year period. They were able to demonstrate the clear correlation between the development of diabetes and rates of exposure to antibiotics; in fact, they showed that **risk for type 2 diabetes was increased by 53% in people who took antibiotics**. In the study abstract, researchers wrote:

> *"There is now mounting evidence… suggesting that antibiotics may drive changes in insulin sensitivity, glucose tolerance, lipid deposition, and energy harvesting potential by altering the gut microbiota composition."*[4]

Antibiotics are also known to increase the permeability of the gut lining, opening up the doorway for disease development. This is commonly called *leaky gut*, and it is this process whereby macromolecules of food and bacteria pass through to the bloodstream resulting in systemic inflammation, insulin spikes and the possible development of autoimmune conditions. According to a paper published in *Gut* in 2006, many diseases, including type 1 diabetes and Crohn's, have a similar disease process where the gut "leaks" an environmental pathogen (toxin) into the bloodstream that causes an abnormal immune reaction in the host. (I go into more detail on this in the *Leaky Gut* section later in this chapter on page 25.)

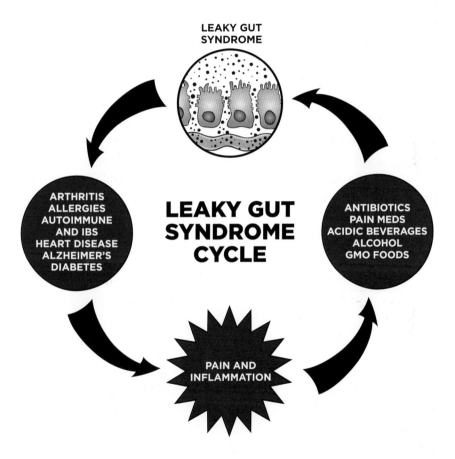

The crux of this is that an increase in gut permeability is a requirement for disease expression.[5]

Are antibiotics evil? No, I don't think so. One must certainly appreciate that antibiotics have indeed saved countless lives throughout the last century; it is our unwitting misuse of them that has caused such dire consequences across the world. First, the general population has drastically reduced the diversity of healthy microbiota in their gut. And then to add insult to injury, our overuse of antibiotics has led to the development of resistant strains of microbes (or bacteria), causing "superbugs." This is a situation where the bugs we're trying to kill become "smarter" than the drugs we're trying to kill them with.

The website for the World Health Organization, www.who.int, describes the situation as follows:

> *"Antimicrobial resistance threatens the effective prevention and treatment of an ever-increasing range of infections caused by bacteria, parasites, viruses, and fungi. It is an increasingly serious threat to global public health that requires action across all government sectors and society. Antimicrobial resistance is present in all parts of the world. New resistance mechanisms emerge and spread globally."* [6]

A British inquiry into antimicrobial resistance found that seven hundred thousand people per year are dying as a result of resistant infections. That same project found that by 2050, if we have not fixed the problem, ten **million** people would die per year![7] Just think, we would no longer be able to perform C-sections, heart surgeries, ER medicine, or re-constructive surgery, all of which rely on antibiotics!

Microbes are able to achieve resistance through "horizontal gene transfer." They are able to "lend and swap" genetic traits so as best to survive any given environment, hence their ability to develop resistance to medications. This is exemplified by a microbe called *Zobellia*, a marine-seaweed dwelling critter who "lends" its genes to Japanese people's microbes so that they can digest seaweeds. It's a trade-off—the host immune system attacks the *Zobellia* in return for borrowing the ability to digest seaweed.

Antibiotic resistance is a serious situation and has inspired Hollywood to produce movies like *Contagion, I Am Legend*, and *Inferno* to depict the potential horrors of a world where infections wipe out populations. These may just be movies for now, but unless we take the threat of microbes spiraling out of control seriously, we are in for a very interesting future.

> Nature is intelligent, seemingly more intelligent than any medicines we create. Until we acknowledge this fact, we'll always be in a health crisis.

Antimicrobial resistance is so dire now that pharmaceutical companies are no longer investing in creating new antibiotics, due to a poor forecast profit model: i.e., no one will buy antibiotics if they don't work. Big Pharma is now focusing on engineering artificial probiotics to assist in disease management, literally creating mutant microbes with specific traits like the ability to kill cancerous cells. What we seem to be discounting here, though, is that every single human being has an immune system which is capable of keeping them well, and many cultures thrive without the use of antibiotics and medicine, such as the Hunzas, Masai, and Okinawans. These cultures may provide more than just test subjects in the future, with interest now growing in the application of their microbiome samples in western populations.

For 80 years we have over-used antibiotics and are now paying the price dearly. Nature is intelligent, seemingly more intelligent than any medicines we create. Until we acknowledge this fact, we'll always be in a health crisis.

Who knows, maybe the coming situation will force us to look at better ways of preventing illness through education and nutrition as opposed to finding new methods of treatment.

There is numerous research to show that probiotics, or beneficial bacteria, have a suppressive effect on pathogenic bacteria and seem to act like natural antibiotics in many cases. Dr. Martin Blaser, author of *Missing Microbes*, has also pointed out that we are shifting into an age where strains of microbes that have coevolved with humans are at risk of being wiped out through the overuse of antibiotics. He gives the example of H. pylori, commonly known as the "stomach ulcer bug." In low concentrations, H. pylori has been shown to modulate appetite and may even be involved with "training" the immune system of the host.[8] But as I explain in the next section, *Quorum Sensing*, H. pylori, when *not kept under control by good bacteria,* can cause negative issues in the gastrointestinal environment.

Quorum Sensing

Microbes are very basic little creatures. They are very small (often single-celled) organisms with only primitive features. Microbe John can't swim along in your gut over to microbe Sally and ask what's going on, so to speak. Thus, microbes have developed a system by which they can actually *read* information about their environment. This form of communication is called *quorum sensing* and it is an important idea to wrap your head around.

Basically, microbes release tiny little molecules called *metabolites* into their environment which can be picked up and read by other microbes in the same environment. Let's use a human analogy. These metabolites are like breadcrumbs; the more breadcrumbs in an environment, the more people you can assume live there. If the breadcrumbs come from paleo bread instead of wondrously white bread, you might be able to guess a little about the type of people in that environment. This is kind of how microbes work in determining what is happening in their environment—they monitor the action of these metabolites to get an idea of what's up.

> You can detox the body all you like, but at some point you need to help the body detox itself!

This system is very important because *microbial DNA expression will change according to the environment the microbes find themselves in.* Bonnie Bassler, molecular biologist, explains how this "chemical language" lets microbes coordinate defense and mount attacks. For instance, H. pylori is a microbe which was commonly thought of as "bad" due to its implications in stomach ulcers. However, Dr. Martin Blaser has shown its potential to train the immune system and regulate appetite. So what's going on?

It is actually the *amount of H. pylori* in the body that determines the influence it has! Little amounts of it may contribute positively to the body, while too much of it may contribute negatively! This is because the H. pylori reads the environment through *quorum sensing,* and when it senses that there are no inhibitors (like probiotics) in place to stop it from proliferating (a goal of all organisms), different genes are switched on, causing it to proliferate and affect the human body in a different way. How interesting is that?

This very important process should put into perspective our idea of "good and bad" bacteria. On both sides of the spectrum, whether complimentary or conventional medicine, practitioners are guilty of *attacking* "bad bugs," when the goal should be maintaining an *overall balance of beneficial microbes in the environment.* This is most important because the healthy populations of *good bugs* help keep the "*bad bugs*" in check!

You can detox the body all you like, but at some point you need to help the body detox itself!

Strong antibiotics or antimicrobial herbs can have their place as an intervention, but the misuse of this approach is not of benefit to the host until we put in place controls which will keep the gut environment healthy over time. Such controls include a healthy diet and a steady intake of probiotic bacteria.

One of the biggest challenges we now face is that science still doesn't know exactly what a "healthy microbiome" looks like. We have manipulated and changed the average person's microbiome so much that it is very hard to determine an optimal one. This is why researchers have begun to look at people from ancient cultures who have not undergone antibiotic treatment as a resource for microbiome research. Recently I traveled to Namibia to conduct some of this research for my documentary *The Gut Movie*, and it was a fascinating experience!

One of the key markers it seems of these ancient tribes is *microbiome diversity*. The Hunzas for instance, who live in pristine areas of the Himalayas, show populations of gut bugs that are vastly wider in diversity to those typically found in the west. Considering that some Hunza are reported to live up to 120 years, and we now the importance of gut health in disease and the aging process, perhaps it is worth examining their gut microbiome.[9] [10]

A potential advancement in our approach to re-establishing microbiome balance for populations in the west may be to literally harvest the poo of these tribes and implant it in individuals over here. This process is proving to be incredibly promising, *however* the complex interplay of gut bugs and the immune system, in conjunction with our diet and lifestyle, still leaves us quite perplexed. Until we understand this process more, expect fecal matter transplants (FMTs) to remain as an "alternative" treatment method.

We've been very clinical about destroying many of the microbes living inside us and not surprisingly we now have a growing population of patients who are experiencing significant health challenges! The cumulative research suggests that an imbalanced microbiome leads to a plethora of health issues, one of which is increased intestinal permeability, commonly known as *leaky gut*.

Leaky Gut

Let's explain leaky gut with a simple analogy.

Picture a screen window. An effective screen lets wonderfully fresh air into your home while keeping out flies, birds, and other undesirable things. But if you've got holes and tears in your screen, some of those undesirables can make it into the home and cause stress. Your intestinal lining is like this screen window.

> *"The intestinal barrier that separates the luminal contents from the systemic circulation is, incredibly, only one cell thick! This extends from the esophagus to the anus. That means that we are dependent on a one cell layer, as well as the connections between these single cells, to carefully screen what is taken in [to the bloodstream] and what is excluded."*
>
> *—David Perlmutter, MD*[11]

The intestinal lining is one-cell thick so that it can let in all the nutrition your cells need to function optimally: vitamins, minerals, trace elements, fatty acids, and more. The problem is if your intestinal lining has increased permeability (or holes, thus a leaky gut). Larger particles of food that would normally move down through your intestines instead move into the bloodstream. Your cells do not recognize these larger molecules, and your immune system reacts by attacking those foreign particles as if they are invaders! Through a process called *molecular mimicry* the body can get confused and start attacking itself, potentially leading to the development of autoimmune disorders like Hashimoto's Thyroiditis and rheumatoid arthritis.[12]

bacteria
 pathogens
 fatty acids
 vitamins & minerals
 glucose
amino acids (protein)

HEALTHY GUT

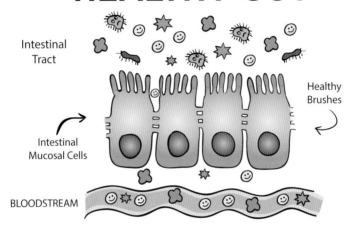

Intestinal Tract

Healthy Brushes

Intestinal Mucosal Cells

BLOODSTREAM

LEAKY GUT
(GI Inflammation)

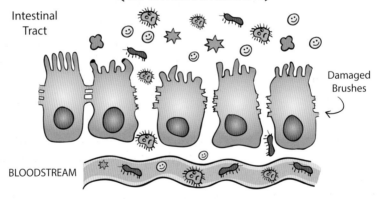

Intestinal Tract

Damaged Brushes

BLOODSTREAM

Systemic Inflammation • Immune System Issues • Food Intolerances • Poor Health

This constant bombardment triggers the immune system to react, resulting in a level of low-grade inflammation throughout the body, which underlies all sorts of health issues from high insulin levels, lowered immunity, and adrenal fatigue. One of the primary roles of the liver is to filter the body's blood supply, and if we want to make that task easy for the liver, we need to reduce the amount of "junk" moving into the bloodstream. This is why short-term liver detox programs are so inadequate for long-term health!

You can detox the liver all you like, *but until you seal up the intestinal wall to prevent non-nutrients from constantly moving into the bloodstream, it'll continue to become toxic.*

> You can detox the liver all you like, but until you seal up the intestinal wall to prevent non-nutrients from constantly moving into the bloodstream, it'll continue to become toxic.

Liver detoxes can be extremely beneficial, but in most instances it is more important to heal the gut lining to prevent liver toxification (from filtering those toxins from the bloodstream) in the first place. Once the gut is sealed properly, the liver can be detoxified by using herbs such as milk thistle, dandelion, and turmeric. Strong antioxidant formulas with a cocktail of botanical and individual antioxidants may also be used.

A leaky gut also allows certain metabolic products to move into the bloodstream and cause health issues. One such product is *lipopolysaccharide (LPS)*, which has been implicated in numerous conditions such as Alzheimer's disease.[13] Even beneficial microbes can move into the bloodstream and cause an immune response, meaning the lining of the gut needs to be healed before some microbes can be ingested (more on that later).

Lipopolysaccharide (LPS): Also known as lipoglycans and endotoxins, lipopolysaccharides (LPS) are complex molecules containing both lipid and polysaccharide parts composed of O-antigen, outer core and inner core joined by a covalent bond; they are found in almost all Gram-negative bacteria and act as extremely strong stimulators of innate or natural immunity in species ranging from insects to humans.

Microbes from Birth

Microbes are like your immune system's personal trainers. By keeping microbes in balance within your body, you're sending them off every day to boxing practice, martial arts, and meditation school.

This happens directly after birth in fact when, as microbiologist John Ellerman shares, *segmented filamentous bacteria* "go in and set up shop" in the host, temporarily dampening the infant's fledgling immune system so that when Mom's bacteria is introduced, they will slowly be recognized as "native" microbes, rather than be attacked and turfed out as invaders.[15]

> "The immune system undergoes major development during infancy and is highly related to the microbes that colonize the intestinal tract."
> —Josef Neu, MD and Jona Rushing, MD[14]

This initial microbial delivery system from mother to infant will then go on to form the template inner ecosystem for that infant's life. Remember that it is Mom's bacteria which inoculate her baby because presumably, these bacteria are suited to (or) come from Mom's environment and food supply and enable the infant to thrive in its new environment. How clever is nature?

"Each kind of bacterium has its own way of affecting the immune system. Some species have been observed to make our immune system more tolerant, for example, by causing more peace-loving, mediatory immune cells to be produced, or by affecting our cells in a similar way to cortisone and other anti-inflammatory drugs."
—Giulia Enders, Microbiologist[16]

This point is also emphasized when we note the data that shows children born via C-section have higher rates of immune-related illnesses.[17] C-section rates in the US rose almost 50% from 1998 to 2011, and we are now seeing around one third of all children being delivered into the world this way. In Australia, rates have risen from 18% in 1991 to 32% in 2015—the World Health Organization says that no region in the world has an excuse to exceed a 10-15% C-section rate.[18]

"Two new HRP studies show that when C-section rates rise towards 10% across a population, the number of maternal and newborn deaths decreases. When the rate goes above 10%, there is no evidence that mortality rates improve."
—World Health Organization[19]

This should be receiving much attention, especially when we consider the initial inoculation process is missed and as a result baby's immune system is compromised. Our drastic haste to deliver babies via C-section in modern times is having significant consequences on the health status of our population and will have future economic repercussions, too.

Recently I became an uncle, and hearing how my brother and sister-in-law had to "fight" with the doctor to ensure a natural birth was interesting. Luckily, they had some excellent midwives who were able to help them stay in control of the situation. Remember that if you are in such a situation, the final decision is always yours.

> *"They might end up with bacteria from Nurse Suzy's right thumb, from the florist who sold Daddy that congratulatory bunch of flowers, or from Grandad's dog."*
> — *Giulia Enders, Microbiologist.*[21]

When a baby moves through Mom's birth canal he/she picks up bacteria that "inoculates" the bodily system. This is like planting seeds in a garden. These bacteria, many of them *Bifidobacteria*, go in and form the basis for baby's inner ecosystem or the microbiome the baby will have for the rest of his/her life! These beneficial microbes then feed upon the indigestible components of Mom's milk, growing and multiplying until they firmly establish themselves. Without these microbes entering the system (like in a C-section delivery), baby may become intolerant to Mom's milk and miss out on the immunological "boot camp" created by these beneficial microbes for the developing immune system. Baby will also have an increased risk of obesity later in life and will take months to establish a healthy microbiome, if at all, as he or she will miss out on the beneficial gut microbes from Mom and may gather microbes elsewhere.[20]

Importantly, if a baby is born naturally but then given antibiotics (a very common situation especially if any inflammatory markers are registered), his/her microbiome will also be compromised.

Of course, C-sections aren't evil and can indeed be life-saving, but if we are to acknowledge the information we now know about the importance of the birthing process in creating a healthy microbiome, then we must take care to inoculate babies born via C-section.

This is why the process of "seeding" has become more popular. Some new mums actually soak a cloth in their vaginal fluid and manually pass this on to their little infants—a stark example of the importance in establishing a healthy inner ecosystem for all women *before* they give birth to a child. Studies have shown that probiotics taken vaginally during pregnancy helped to balance the vaginal microflora that is then passed onto the newborn baby.[22]

I would also suggest speaking with your doctor about keeping pharmaceutical-grade probiotic supplements on hand which contain strains of beneficial bacteria for infants should a C-section result. For instance, studies have shown that administration of Lactobacillus bacteria to C-section babies reduces the risk of developing allergies.[23] Moms, if concerned (after consulting with their practitioner), may be advised to put probiotic strains on the nipple before breastfeeding to pass on these beneficial microbes to baby. Again, it's not about making anyone feel guilty for conducting a C-section, but rather about objectively acknowledging the implications of doing so and working toward correcting any potential imbalances which may result.

It is of extreme importance during the developmental years for children to have a healthy, well-functioning microbiome.

According to Dr. Natasha Campbell-McBride, author and creator of the Gut and Psychology Syndrome or GAPS diet, the microbiome is the determining factor behind whether or not a child functions optimally or goes on to develop conditions such as autism and ADHD. She says that when the microbiome and gut become a source of *toxicity* as opposed to a source of *nutrition*, the developing brain of the young child is compromised.

> *"That usually happens in the second year of life in children who were breast fed because breastfeeding provides a protection against this abnormal gut flora. In children who were not breastfed, I see the symptoms of autism developing in the first year of life. So, breastfeeding is crucial to protect these children."* [24]

Dr. Campbell McBride points out that it's in those first two years of life that the brain matures, learns communication skills and instinctive behaviors. Sensory information being sent from the gut to the brain is disrupted and compromised due to the abnormal microbiota in the gut, affecting the neurology of the child.

> *"If the child's brain is clogged with toxicity, the child misses that window of opportunity for learning and starts developing autism depending on the mixture of toxins, depending on how severe the whole condition is, and how severely abnormal the gut flora is in the child."*[25]

Scientists are now considering the microbiome as a key player in modulating an immune response to a vaccine in a human.[26] For instance, in "third world" populations where poor sanitation can lead to imbalanced microbiomes, rates of positive response to vaccinations are reduced. We also need to consider the effects of vaccines on the microbiome. Whether you are pro or anti-vaccine, we must acknowledge that the presence of certain additives, preservatives and adjuncts in vaccinations may indeed disrupt the delicate ecology of the microbiome. Vaccines contain ingredients like aluminum because these substances irritate the immune system. This stimulates it to mount an immune response to the virus/bacteria introduced with the vaccine. The body then develops antibodies against the bacteria or virus.[27]

"Just as today the kids are lining up for the vaccines, in the future, maybe the kids are going to be drinking certain organisms so that we can replace the ones that they've lost."[28]

—*Dr. Martin Blaser*

Dr. Natasha Campbell-McBride points out that vaccinations were originally developed for children with *healthy* immune systems (healthy microbiomes). She says that children with Gut and Psychology Syndrome (imbalanced microbiomes) are not fit to be vaccinated and when we consider the fact that *most children* these days do have some sort of imbalanced microbiome, this translates to a very small number of children who are eligible for vaccines (according to Mcbride's criteria).

"It's a matter of the last straw breaking the camel's back. So if the child is damaged enough, the vaccine can provide that last straw. But if it doesn't provide that last straw in a particular child, then it will get the child closer to the breaking point."[29]

One must also recognize the fact that the viruses and bacteria that we receive in vaccines *are almost all synthetically created*. So this means that we are trying to inoculate against naturally occurring diseases with unnaturally occurring microbes. Understand that it is very difficult for us to determine the exact effects of these vaccines on each host's immune system and microbiome. Dr. Suzanne Humphries writes in *Dissolving Illusions:*

> *"Even modern smallpox vaccines do not actually contain cowpox or smallpox virus but a human/animal hybrid agent that never existed in nature until the era of vaccination."*[30]

This is certainly not an argument against vaccination. It is not my place to mount such an argument. Yet I do want to encourage you to be aware of the implications of vaccinations *particularly on the developing microbiome and immune system of a child*. You as an individual *should be very informed* about all the decisions you make regarding your wellbeing. You alone must weigh the risk and benefits of vaccinations. Do not be afraid to ask your doctor about the vaccines he/she recommends—it is their job to inform you about the potential side effects and benefits of such interventions.

Blindly submitting to any sort of medical procedure or intervention, (especially when there is a strong financial incentive for its application[31]) would be downright illogical. As parents, uncles, aunties, brothers and sisters, you have a right to be informed before you make choices regarding your own or your family's health. As always, that choice should be yours to make.

Okay, moving on.

It may also be the case that babies are born prematurely due to microbes, as Josef Neu, MD and Jona Rushing, MD write:

> *"While the paradigm has been that babies' intestines are sterile until birth, recent work found a microbial community already dwelling in the meconium of some babies born*

prematurely. It has also been shown that amniotic fluid of mothers with preterm labor contains a large and diverse spectrum of bacterial rDNA. While a baby is in utero, it typically swallows 400 to 500 milliliters of amniotic fluid per day at term, and the hypothesis that intra-amniotic infection is the driving force behind preterm labor is one being widely studied in obstetrics."[32]

One of the most significant approaches we could take for long-term health of the world's population is to ensure that mothers have a strong, healthy microbiome to pass onto their child. By taking a conscious, holistic, and gentle approach to pregnancy, this can certainly be achieved!

Don't forget that males have to be on board, too, as their microbes heavily influence sperm health, and they physically pass their bacteria onto Mom and her birth canal during intercourse. For those concerned with the health of their skin biome in these areas, swabbing the reproductive area around the groin and testicles with apple cider vinegar and probiotic strains can be a good idea (yeah, seriously). For vaginal infections, where often there is an overgrowth of yeast involved, try douching with apple cider vinegar or inserting a Lactobacillus probiotic via an enema kit.

Microbial Influence

Ever known someone who has had their appendix removed? Scientists are now postulating that the appendix is the body's last and final reserve of good bacteria, but when there are no good bacteria left it becomes infected, inflamed, and must be removed. This is evidenced in "germ-free" mice (a mouse with no microbiome), which studies show develop swollen appendices alongside abnormal eating behavior and poor immune function. However, scientists were able to reverse these negative effects of appendicitis by shrinking the appendices down to normal size and normalizing their eating behavior with the application of specific strains of bacteria.[33]

In most cases, it seems that probiotic microbes exert a suppressive effect on pathogenic microbes. In a fascinating study conducted at Washington University, researchers developed "germ-free" mice and were able to determine their weight outcomes simply by changing the type of bacteria they were inoculated with. Mice inoculated with bacteria from a lean person stayed lean, while mice inoculated with bacteria from an obese person got obese. Importantly, both groups of mice were eating the same diet. Upon allowing the mice to group together however, whereby the mice shared bacteria by eating each other's poo, the obese mice became lean, too![34] This means you may want to take care when selecting the partner with whom you share microbes, but it also suggests that beneficial bacteria are able to create an environment where they can thrive and suppress potentially detrimental bacteria.

Having a good amount of probiotics in place within the gastrointestinal tract will naturally create an environment that favors their proliferation. Probiotics help modulate the acid/alkaline balance of your intestine, and, via chemical signaling through the vagus nerve, will literally tell your brain to consume certain foods. They will sometimes even "attack" pathogenic microbes—all with the intention of perpetuating their own existence inside you!

In the birth canal for instance we see a good example of a species of beneficial bacteria modulating the environment in its favor. Lactobacillus bacteria make up around half of the bacteria occupying the birth canal. They produce lactic acid which in turn creates an environment where only those microbes that enjoy a lactic acid environment can set up home.[35] This is like screening everybody who wants to come to the party and making sure they pass the "acid test" at the door.

Exploring how weight is influenced by the microbiome may be a more complex process than simply "obese" microbes harvesting more calories from food than their "lean" counterparts. Pathogenic microbial infections may actually hinder the thyroid gland, causing it to produce fewer thyroid hormones and resulting in metabolic disruption (more fat storage).[36] One must also realize that having excess fat tissue in itself is conducive to an inflammatory state. Far from being an inert storage facility, your fat cells are covered in healthy immune cells (*Tregs*) which help them communicate with your immune system. If someone becomes obese, the fat cells can change. The Treg cells, which normally dampen inflammation, disappear, allowing inflammation to go unchecked, which results in a metabolic environment conducive to storing extra weight.[37]

Tregs: Regulatory T cells, formerly known as suppressor T cells, that maintain order in the immune system, maintain tolerance to self-antigens, and prevent autoimmune disease.

Your microbes constantly communicate with your Treg cells. So, could it be that the "obese" microbes actually trigger the Tregs to become inert or disappear, resulting in a highly efficient fat-storage facility? Or is the fat itself to blame? We'll certainly learn more in the future.

The Gut-Brain Connection

The gut-brain connection is something that's been talked about for thousands of years ever since Hippocrates said, "all disease begins in the gut." However, it's only been in the last two decades, if that, in which science has provided strong evidence of the positive effect which probiotics and improved gut health can have on neurological function.

The gut-brain connection, the communication between the gut and the brain via the vagus nerve, has been firmly established and scientists are now stating that the gut nervous system may have even more neurons than the brain! This gives much weight to the idea that your gut and digestive system, as we've learned throughout this book, is far more than just a passageway for food.

Who would have thought that the microbes in our gut could have an influence on our decision-making?

In animal studies, mice manually infected with toxoplasma (a parasite typically found in cats) subsequently lost their fear of cats. Extraordinarily, even after being treated for the infection with an antibiotic, the fearless behavior towards cats remained, suggesting a permanent effect from the infection on the brain![38]

According to the latest science, your gut microbes have a large influence on how you think. Around 95% of *serotonin*, for example is actually manufactured in the gut![39] An important neurotransmitter, serotonin, when lacking, is attributed to the development of depression. Gut microbes also have a large influence on the levels of *BDNF (Brain Derived Neurotrophic Factor)* and *GABA (Gamma Amino Butyric Acid)* in the neurological system, further influencing brain health. Both of these "brain chemicals" have been shown to have positive effects on our neurological function. BDNF optimizes synaptic plasticity which aids learning and memory retention. Interestingly, it is found in highest amounts in the areas of the brain that control hunger, thirst, and metabolism! GABA on the other hand, is responsible for calming nerve transmission and activity within the brain, allowing you to deal with stressful situations by thinking calmly.[40] These are just two examples of how healthy microbes in the gut aid brain function.

Serotonin: Serotonin, the body's "feel good" neurotransmitter, is involved in the transmission of nerve impulses. It is manufactured in the brain and the intestines. The majority of the body's serotonin can be found in the gastrointestinal (GI) tract.

BDNF (Brain Derived Neurotrophic Factor): BDNF is a protein that influences brain function as well as the peripheral nervous system. BDNF builds and maintains the brain circuits which allow the signals of neurons to travel. It is an important factor in memory and mood.

GABA (Gamma Amino Butyric Acid): GABA is a neurotransmitter of the central nervous system that inhibits excitatory responses. GABA contributes to motor control, vision, and many other cortical functions. It also regulates anxiety.

With so much evidence (both scientific and anecdotal) supporting the theory that probiotic supplementation and correcting gut function can improve our mental health, how are we still so out of balance?

Remember that nature always strives for balance. It can be argued that extreme states of depression, anxiety, and mood swings are not intended in nature, but rather the result of an *im*balance somewhere in the body. Those struggling with mental health challenges should certainly request from their doctor or practitioner some sort of gut-health test or at least a standardized questionnaire which may provide some insight when a microbiome test is not available.

One cannot ignore our unwitting use of antibiotics over the past 80 years as one factor underlying such an imbalance. The unfortunate thing about antibiotics, as previously written, is that we now have a population whose microbiomes are completely and, in many cases, permanently altered. We don't really know what an *ideal* microbiome is anymore—all we do know is that ours have changed completely since the use of antibiotics and we may even be seeing a rise in mental illness, in part, as a result of poor gut health.

Another factor in the gut-brain connection, it seems, is the management of inflammation by the actions of gut microbes and the immune system. Our gut bugs are literally talking with our immune cells, teaching them from the first time you enter the world how to behave cordially and appropriately. Naturally, if our gut bugs are imbalanced, we can experience numerous immunological challenges. This, according to the research, seems to stem from increased intestinal permeability (again, leaky gut). Alongside the macromolecules of food, pathogenic microbes and other such intruders that enter the bloodstream through a permeable gut lining, another molecule appears that is damaging to the brain. That molecule is LPS, which was discussed previously in the *Leaky Gut* section. LPS has been found in extremely high levels in Alzheimer's disease and is known to cause neuron damage in the brain.[41]

LPS and brain inflammation may be extremely instrumental in the development of such mental illnesses as depression, anxiety, and mood swings as the brain becomes less capable of processing information. In fact, this has been supported in studies where researchers have administered probiotics to mice and noted striking differences in their behavior. Mice who receive probiotic treatment and are then subjected to stressful situations release less of the stress hormone cortisol (than mice who don't receive the probiotic) and behaviorally appear calmer.[42] Further, this experiment has been replicated in humans with similar results showing that probiotic treatment regularly reduces qualitative anxiety scores.[43]

A study published in 2016 on the use of probiotic treatment on Alzheimer's patients showed actual reversals of blood indicators associated with Alzheimer's and improvements in mental function for patients using probiotic treatment, while the control group (not taking any probiotics) continued to worsen in those same markers![44]

These results are significant because, normally, most research into Alzheimer's looks at the possibility of only reducing the rate of cognitive decline, *not actually reversing it.*

Dr. Natasha Campbell-McBride goes as far as to say that autism is the manifestation of a gut which has become a source of toxicity instead a source of nutrition during developmental years. According to her, if the condition is treated early enough, the autistic symptoms can be reversed. This opinion is supported by research showing that autistic children often have different gut microbes from non-autistic children, and in particular have higher levels of microbes like E. coli and clostridia.[45]

So, what does all this mean?

It means that if we want to experience great mental as well as physical health, then considering an approach which targets the gut is a good move.

By taking a sensible, long-term approach that includes a regimen of probiotics and a whole-foods, high-fiber diet, like I have outlined in this book, people can expect more ease in attaining a balanced neurology.

As science continues to uncover the role of the microbiome in overall health and begins pinpointing the specific bacterial bugs that may underlie specific diseases, we can expect huge improvements and changes in the symptom-based approach of western medicine. We may even see a rise in the number of holistic psychiatrists who prescribe specific strains of probiotics to their patients for some conditions in addition or instead of the litany of psychotropic drugs administered today.

Allergies Rhinitis (Hay Fever)

Hay fever is an increased sensitivity/irritation of the mucous membranes of the gastro-intestinal system and *subsequent* further irritation of the olfactory and oropharynx mucous membranes. This can be caused by an excessive histamine response in the body from the *degranulation* of certain immune cells.

In an era when the symptom-based approach to disease has quite literally spiraled out of control, examining and focusing on the root cause of hay fever is a much smarter approach for long-term cessation of the condition. On the basis of the research it can be said quite confidently that the regular intake of probiotics throughout the year (as opposed to only during allergy season) is our best option for the prevention of hay fever symptoms.

A specific probiotic called *Lactobacillus rhamnosus* (LGG) has been shown to down-regulate the immune cell degranulation process that leads to hay fever symptoms.[46] This is an important indicator that probiotic-immune cell interaction may be at the root of allergic response.

Degranulation: Degranulation is the loss of secretory vesicles called granules in certain cells. It is used by several different cells involved in the immune system.

A systematic review published on the topic in 2015 examined 23 prominent studies in the area of probiotics and allergic rhinitis, covering a total of 1,919 participants. The researchers looked mainly at the subjective quality of life as reported in questionnaires given the participants throughout the studies. The review found that of the 23 studies, 17 showed significant improvements for participants taking probiotics. That is, for 74% of the studies, allergy sufferers reported big improvements in quality of life while taking probiotics compared to those who didn't.[47]

Food Allergies

As we've spoken about throughout this book, the immune system is intricately linked with the microbes in your gastrointestinal system. According to experts, leaky gut can often be the root cause of food allergies. The constant bombardment of undigested, macromolecules of food passing through the intestinal lining and into the bloodstream triggers an immune response within the body. This response is similar to how the body reacts to any consistent, foreign invader. The immune system develops specific antibodies to quickly and efficiently nullify the invader, in this case the offending food particles. This results in an often-hyperactive immune response, where natural food products can cause an immediate and intense allergic reaction.

By harnessing the gut-restorative power of probiotics, one may be able to restore integrity to the gut lining and stop this phenomenon from reoccurring.[48] Over the long term, the restorative power of a gut-nourishing diet and subsequent improvement of the microbiome may have a similar effect.

In a fascinating study, researchers from the Murdoch Children's Research Institute in Australia were able to drastically reduce allergic responses to peanuts by administering probiotic therapy! In a place-bo-controlled study, over 60 peanut-allergic children were either given a dose of a specific probiotic, *Lactobacillus rhamnosus* together with peanut protein in slowly increasing amounts or a placebo over 18 months.

Incredibly, researchers found that over 80% of the children who received the oral immunotherapy treatment were able to tolerate pea-nuts at the end of the trial, compared to less than 4% of the placebo group. This is 20 times higher than the natural rate of resolution for peanut allergy.[49]

The research strongly suggests that allergies have deep roots in the balance (or lack thereof) of our gut microbes. So, if you do suffer from them, a gut-centered approach may be a wise strategy moving forward.

Digestion

When I speak at events and ask who in the audience thinks their digestion is optimal, around 5% of the audience put their hands up. That's not a good number, especially when we know that good diges-tion is essential to wellbeing. Importantly, this is in a room *where at least 75% of the audience considers their diet to be very healthy!* The diges-tion equation is complex, involving not just our diet, but also our stress levels, *how* we eat, *who* we eat with, and of course the state of our microbiome!

The thing is, *you* aren't really digesting your food anyway, it's the microbiota inside you that digest the food for you.

The saying, "you are what you eat" is only partially correct, because you are only what your body absorbs.

> The saying, "you are what you eat" is only partially correct, because you are only what your body absorbs.

Many people eat healthily, and yet do not absorb what they need from their food.

Enzymes have long been cited as the be-all-end-all substances required for healthy digestion, yet the human body only has a store of 30 different enzymes. Our microbes make up for our shortcomings in this area as the largest producer of enzymes in the entire body. For instance, just one single species, *Bacteroidetes thetaiotaomicron,* contains the potential to make over 260 specific enzymes for breaking down plant fibers.[50]

I picture my microbes as little guys lined up on an assembly line in a factory, waiting to receive big shipments of food from the esophagus. Then they break those packages down into their individual parts and organize them in a sensible order before sending them off to be absorbed into the system. There are some employees who like to eat up some of the prebiotic fibers that come through the factory, but in return they leave behind wonderful nutrients like butyrate which are then sent off for anti-inflammatory duties around the body.[51] There are also some "employees" whose numbers need to be kept in check; things like sugar and alcohol tend to send them out of control.

It's a pretty marvelous set up, the ol' digestive system, and it's certainly something we've taken for granted. In the somewhat cheeky, but equally marvelous book *Gut,* Giulia Enders writes of the intricacies of the gut that we should all know about. Writing about the villi (those finger-like projections lining the small intestine), she says:

"Even greater magnification reveals that each and every one of those cells is itself covered with little protrusions— the microvilli—villi on villi, if you like. The microvilli are in turn covered with a velvety meshwork of countless sugar-based structures that look a little bit like antlers. These are called glycocalyces. If all this, the folds, villi, and the microvilli, were ironed out to a smooth surface, our gut would have to be some seven kilometers in length."[52]

It's this 7km (4.35 miles) of highly absorbent area that is the fundamental reason for the existence of the gut. It allows you to move nutrition from your food into the bloodstream. This is the sole reason for digestion in the first place; to take that apple or cherry, send it along the gastrointestinal tract, and break it down to the molecular level so the micronutrients can be delivered to each and every cell around the body.

The integrity of this process is somewhat fragile—as it relies on the proper functioning of the one-cell-thick membrane surrounding the gut—the gut lining. The fragility of the gut lining is also its greatest strength because this thin membrane allows for maximum absorption of the micronutrients broken down from food—which are required for cell metabolism and functions—keeping the body alive and well. However, this fragility comes at a price, as various factors can increase permeability excessively, allowing unwanted molecules to enter the bloodstream.

This sieve-like process is delicate. Harboring an infection of bad bacteria can compromise the gut lining and thus digestion and nutrient absorption. The "finger-like" villi and the Peyer's patches *between* some of the villi act as receptors for the immune system, communicating back and forth to the immune cells to relay what's going on. If pathogenic bacteria adhere to the Peyer's patches for instance, your resistance to infection is down-regulated and your levels of inflammation are increased. When good bacteria adheres to those patches, the opposite occurs.[53]

If for some reason the intestinal villi and microvilli are damaged, like in the case of classic celiac conditions where the villi become more "stump-like," then we begin to see issues with malabsorption. It becomes difficult for the body to obtain adequate nutrition from food like iron, magnesium, and zinc, thus we end up with deficiencies. Complimentary medicine can be just as guilty as western medicine at "covering up symptoms" in this regard by offering a plain old zinc or iron supplement when the root cause is in the state of the small intestinal villi. There are many people now with fructose malabsorption, amine, and salicylate intolerances, all of whom could potentially overcome these issues just by re-establishing the health of their intestinal villi and gut lining. Sometimes this takes months, even years to occur; it depends on the level of damage within the system.

A similar process may also be causing common digestive conditions such as Crohn's disease. The fungus *Candida tropicalis*, alongside two bacteria called *Escherichia coli* (*E. coli*) and *Serratia marcescens*, may be the culprits according to research. A team of international researchers published a study[54] claiming these three microbes were found in significantly higher amounts in people with Crohn's disease in comparison to healthy individuals.

Furthermore, the same team found that the three species work together in test tubes to produce a biofilm—a thin, slimy layer of microorganisms found in the body that adheres to, among other sites, a portion of the intestines—prompting inflammation and the symptoms known as Crohn's disease.[55]

Stomach Acid

The stomach is normally quite an acidic environment, and this has many distinct advantages, especially when it comes to keeping parasites and nasty bugs at bay. The reality is that parasites abound on most of our food! Consider that daily we eat produce which has been grown in nature, thrown in the back of a truck, and passed from hand to hand. We regularly and unknowingly ingest these parasites, but quite often they are either killed off by the acidic environment of our stomach or they simply pass through the entire system unnoticed.

Just now writing this book, I was just unwittingly licked *in the mouth* by a dog, yet I'm not concerned because I know my stomach acid is probably strong enough to sanitize any potential nasties from the dog. (Oh, pets.)

The high acid content of the stomach acts as a sterilizing agent that protects us from the nastiest of microbes. But when there is not enough acid present (for instance in someone taking acid-blocking drugs), this protective mechanism is undermined.[56] The initial problems with acid reflux often stem from poor food combining, eating too fast, and eating imbalanced meals (too much protein, for instance). Although acid-blockers can provide temporary relief from these symptoms, they actually worsen the gut environment so that you digest food even more poorly and end up at higher risk for infections from parasites and pathogenic bacteria!

Probiotics can modulate this environment so that your hydrochloric acid (HCL) production can be normalized, protecting you from foreign invaders on your food. Himalayan salt and apple cider vinegar have also been used by complimentary practitioners to stimulate hydrochloric acid production. Taking HCL tablets may be necessary in *some* instances, but is best determined by working with your practitioner. However, emphasis should be placed on re-establishing the body's capability to produce HCL internally. Maintaining healthy levels of hydrochloric acid in your stomach will ensure a gut environment which supports beneficial microbes.

Missing Microbes and Fermented Foods

It's been firmly established that traditional cultures have a much wider diversity of microbial residents in their bodies, but where do they get them? Aside from receiving some of them at birth from Mom, people in these cultures are exposed to microbes on a daily basis. These communities place little emphasis on the same standards of cleanliness and sterilization as western cultures, which means they are exposed to a diverse variety of microbes through particles of soil on food and from fermented foods. When I was living with the San in Namibia for my documentary *The Gut Movie*, we ate foods directly from the ground, teeming with dirt! The San do not wash regularly and are always in contact with nature, resulting in their diverse microbiomes.

For thousands of years people have fermented food as a way to preserve edibles for later access when food supply is low. The American Indians, for instance, would bury food underground for years at a time and come back to enjoy it in times of scarcity. The Chinese do this as well; they grow cabbages in the countryside and ferment them for the harsh winters as a readily available food source. Indigenous Australians would gather sour ants, medicinal herbs, and flowers and ferment those into a delicious drink. The Masai of Kenya ferment raw cow's milk, while the Hunzas ferment raw goat's milk! I remember walking the streets of El Salvador on a surf trip and finding the locals with massive containers of kimchi!

We do still have ancient strains of bacteria among us in the west today. The survival and perpetuation of kefir and the SCOBY in kombucha (both discussed in detail in Chapter 8) is testament to their amazing propensity to survive and replicate over time. The scarcity of these foods in the western diet for the past 50 to 80 years has certainly resulted in our microbiome becoming more "sterile" and as a result we are more prone to illness. For the long-term maintenance of your microbiome, fermented foods can be a fantastic tool for you to use every day. (Be sure to check out my online Fermented Foods Mastery course at kalebrock.com.) For those with gut challenges, it is often a good idea to do some gut healing *before* the introduction of fermented foods into the diet. This is to ensure that the gut lining is sealed and does not allow wild bacteria from fermented food into the bloodstream.

To an extent, it may be our obsession with cleanliness that has gotten us to where we are today. The endeavor to "attack" bacteria and "wipe it clean" may be beneficial in some instances, such as in commercial kitchens, but it may not be serving us well in a general health sense. Studies have shown that farm children have healthier immune systems and less disease than "clean" city kids.[57] I remember playing amongst the rocks and dirt and chasing mud crabs on the beach when I was young. I've no doubt those microbes entered my system and hey, I'd go as far as saying maybe they're the reason I love the ocean so much. (That's my excuse; it's a *biological* need.)

Needless to say, rather than removing all microbes from our lives, we should be much more interested in creating an environment, in our homes and bodies, where only the good guys can grow. Now let's show you how to do that.

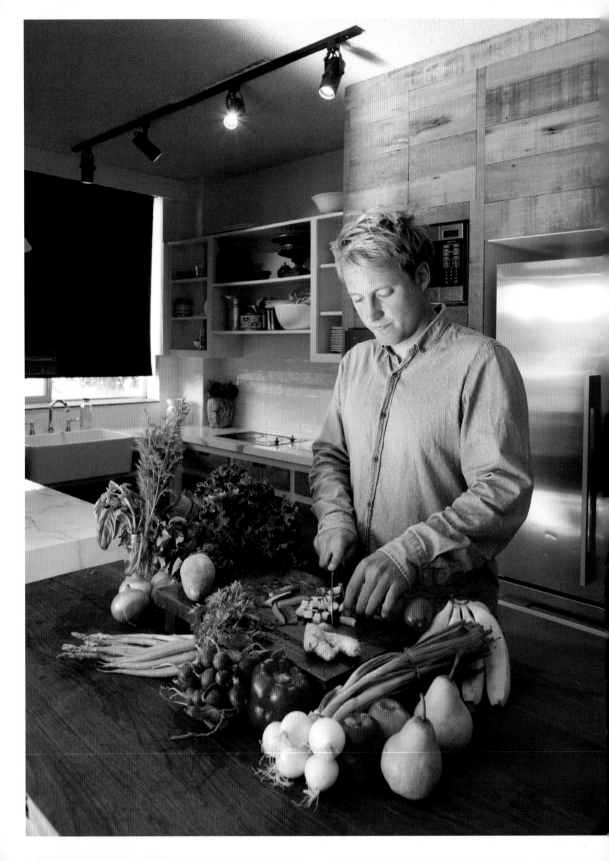

CHAPTER 4

Dietary and Lifestyle Principles
for the GHP

A gut-healing protocol, in order to be effective, needs to address two main things within the GI tract:

1. We need to rebalance the population of microbes and stimulate and encourage the intestinal lining to heal.

2. We need to modify the diet to foster the growth of healthy microbes and utilize certain foods and supplements to heal the gut lining to do this.

Dr. Raphael Kellman, author of *The Microbiome Diet*, suggests the following steps when healing the gut:

- Remove

- Replace

- Reinoculate

- Repair

I would add in the following step:

- Evolve the diet

Functional medicine practitioners share a similar approach.

Weeding—clears out infections of pathogenic microbes and rebalances their numbers.

Seeding—inoculates the gut with probiotic microbes (often using very specific strains depending on the test results of the individual).

Feeding—adopt a wholesome diet with plenty of insoluble fibers which provide fuel for the probiotic microbes.

Both approaches are logical and follow a step-by-step system to healing the gut. These are the fundamental principles on which I have based my Gut Healing Protocol. As always, a healing program *needs to be tailored for the individual.* Each person's microbiome is unique and requires a slightly different method to heal, but the *framework* should always follow the aforementioned principles. Establishing the specifics of your own gut-healing program should be done with a good health practitioner if available—however if you are not suffering from any serious illness, then a general approach often delivers great results.

Remember, it is the ongoing systemic environment that determines the long-term health of the microbiome, which is why we always emphasize a *long-term approach* to health and wellness.

Naturally, in this protocol we focus on ***removing*** inflammatory foods from the diet, such as foods that may fuel a yeast infection. We are also removing pathogenic microbes (or, rather, rebalancing their numbers into non-disease-causing proportions) that may be present. This step is akin to functional medicine's *Weeding* stage. Probiotic supplementation and the use of herbal antimicrobials can be used here.

Inherently as part of the initial steps of a good gut-healing program is the ***replacing*** step. We want to replace the stomach acid and enzymes in your digestive system by using probiotic supplementation, alkalizing your body, and using high-quality enzymatically rich foods such as salads and other vegetables.

Reinoculating (functional medicine's *Seeding*) your gut with beneficial bacteria from probiotic supplements is an extremely important step. In the coming pages, we will cover the intricacies of this.

The GHP outlined in this book will also provide your new healthy microbes with loads of prebiotic rich foods such as carrots, onion, turmeric, beets, and tomatoes so they can begin to establish themselves permanently within your gut. This loading up of fiber-rich foods is the *Feeding* aspect of the functional medicine system.

It is not enough to simply take high doses of probiotic supplements and continue to eat poorly. For long-term wellbeing, it is essential that you adopt a clean, wholesome diet to support your new microbial residents!

If you have a polluted lake. you don't just go ahead and throw a bunch of healthy fish in there, do you? First you clean up the lake, remove all the algae and sludge, reinoculate the lake with healthy fish. and maintain its new level of cleanliness.

Repairing your intestinal lining and microbiome will naturally take place over the 8 weeks on this protocol as we reduce the inflammation in your gut and provide nourishing microbes to help reduce your intestine's "leakiness." Consuming bone broth on a regular basis and supplementing with bovine colostrum and/or Aloe vera will also help to heal the gut epithelium. This, like all the other steps, is essential to establishing *long-term* change in the gastrointestinal tract. (More on this in the following pages.)

Before we go into which foods *are* encouraged on the Gut Healing Protocol, let's look at the foods that most practitioners recommend you eliminate.

Wheat

In his monumental book *Wheat Belly,* Dr. William Davis shatters the myth that the consumption of whole grains, especially wheat and gluten-containing grains, is healthy for the human body. Davis presents a compelling story on the overall inflammatory properties of wheat, which when consumed can lead to obesity, leaky gut syndrome, diabetes, acidosis, accelerated aging, heart disease, neurological issues, and more. He points out in his book that two slices of whole wheat bread can actually raise blood sugar more than two tablespoons of pure sugar—which is alarming when we consider the consequences of fluctuating blood sugar on health and longevity.[58]

One of the main issues with wheat consumption seems to be that we have heavily altered its genetic structure and the subsequent content of gluten proteins over the past few generations. Added to that is the problem of farming in depleted soil, spraying with carcinogenic pesticides, and inappropriately storing the grain, leading to the growth of mold and pathogens.

The inflammatory properties of wheat and gluten in grains have been extensively studied over the past few decades, with researchers such as Professor Alessio Fasano (chief of Pediatric Gastroenterology and Nutrition at MassGeneral Hospital for Children and visiting professor of pediatrics at Harvard Medical School) showing how gluten consumption leads to increased intestinal permeability (leaky gut) in everyone who consumes it *even if they do not have celiac or gluten sensitivity.* He points out that *"for the 2.5 million years of evolution, 99.9% of our species has been gluten-free."*[59] Fasano has shown that gluten stimulates the release of a protein called *zonulin* that modulates the permeability of the gut lining (in this case, increasing it), opening up the doorway for the development of diseases like Hashimoto's, arthritis, and diabetes.

On ABC's *Catalyst* program, *Gluten: A Gut Feeling,* gluten was put under an intense spotlight.

"It [gluten] doesn't have much flavour and, in fact, has very little nutritional value. But you add water, and its unique properties come to light. Gluten is a protein made up of two molecules, glutenin and gliadin, which form an elastic bond in the presence of water. Gluten is what makes dough sticky and flexible. And while it's found naturally in wheat and other grains, bakers often add extra gluten to bread to give it that spongy texture."[60]
—*Dr. Maryanne Demasi, medical journalist.*

Gluten seems to act this way in the digestive tract as well. Thanks to its glue-like properties, gluten may slow digestion, causing irritation and fermentation within the gut, creating an environment not conducive to a healthy microbiome or intestinal lining. If you're interested in healing the gut and your immune system, then it is a must that you get off gluten at least in the short term. The gluten molecule itself is extremely inflammatory and can lead to abnormal immune responses and damage of the organs.

"It triggers an abnormal immune response that leads to damage to a variety of organs. This includes the bowel. This also includes the skin, the joints, the bones, the nervous system, the liver. It's a very systemic condition."[61]
—*Dr. Jason Tye Din, gastroenterologist.*

This inflammatory characteristic of wheat and gluten-containing grains is one of the main reasons we must avoid them if we are to heal our intestinal lining effectively. Dr. Raphael Kellman in his book *The Microbiome Diet* recommends removing **all** inflammatory foods from the diet including gluten, sugar, eggs (more on this later), soy, dairy, trans fats and artificial preservatives so that the gut can heal.

Dr. David Perlmutter in his book *Grain Brain* cites much of this gluten research and focuses on the role of gluten in neurological health, summarizing that it can have acute effects on behavior and mood and chronic effects on the physiology of the brain itself. Dr. Perlmutter advocates a diet that is low in carbohydrate, moderate in proteins and high in healthy fats, very similar to the protocol in this book.[62]

Added to the disastrous effects of gluten, wheat is considered a very *mycotoxic food*, meaning it exacerbates or contains pathogenic molds or fungus. Dave Asprey (of *Bulletproof Exec*) has championed the anti-mycotoxin approach to eating, which is an approach that has a solid scientific basis; much research has been done on the implications of extrinsic and intrinsic mycotoxins. It's interesting because in farming circles it is very common to find mold growth in conjunction with stored grain. I remember working on a farm in outback Australia cleaning out silos filled with wheat and finding mold everywhere! I came out of each silo with an irritating, ugly rash all over my arms and all I could think was, *people eat this stuff?*

There is an argument that ancient forms of wheat (e.g., einkorn wheat) may still be appropriate for consumption. This might be true of ancient cultures with uncompromised and adapted microbiomes, however it remains a good idea to avoid even these strains of wheat while on the Gut Healing Protocol or a gut-nourishing diet. The inflammatory nature of grains (simply because they contain substances designed by nature to protect them from being consumed) is something the compromised gut can do without.

It may well be that there are other substances in wheat that the human body is sensitive to, but regardless of the mechanistic functions of wheat in the body, in order for the gut to heal we need to cut it out. Going gluten free is fantastic when replaced by the more fibrous vegetables and fruits. It does not mean buying the gluten free bread and pastries as a replacement. Down the line, it may be that traditionally fermented gluten-containing grains do work for your unique body, but ensure your gut is healed for at least a year before introducing these foods. The research is still out on wheat, but unfortunately it is not particularly impressive, especially when it comes to ensuring the health of the gastro-intestinal tract.

Dairy

In the east of Africa lives a tribe of people called the Masai. These healthy people live an active, happy, and largely disease-free life in their ever-shrinking territory. They eat a predominantly dairy-based diet, around 85% in fact. Milk is collected from their revered cattle and allowed to sit at room temperature in large pots. The naturally-occurring bacteria in the milk break down the proteins and sugars, turning the milk sour and curdy and making it easily digestible by the *bacteria* in the Masai people's digestive tracts. The Masai thrive on this diet.

So why tell you this? To illustrate the point that there are no black and white solutions when it comes to diet, and that just because there are "poor" versions of dairy (namely processed), does not mean that all dairy is somehow evil or bad as a food or industry. One of the amazing dairy products that is important for health is bovine colostrum, or mother's first milk. Full of antibodies and immune-boosting properties, it is an excellent healer of the gut with numerous other health benefits, too. We will be embracing the benefits of colostrum in this protocol as a supplemental food.

That being said though, dairy, *in general* is not a food that is included on the GHP. But what about the Masai? The dairy that the Masai consume is raw and biofermented, *and* the Masai microbiome is well-suited to such a diet after thousands of years of adaptation. These factors are key in distinguishing the difference between their dairy and our dairy. The milk, cheese, cream, and other products that we have access to in the west (for the most part) have been pasteurized (heated to kill off all bacteria), often homogenized, and contains trace amounts of chemicals including antibiotics and pesticides from the feed the cows live on, and BPA from the plastic containers it is stored in. This is far removed from the dairy products consumed by the Masai or even by us in the old days.

Dr. Raphael Kellman paints the picture well when he says that even the tiniest amounts of skim milk used in coffee can set off a systemic immune reaction to inflammatory molecules from milk as they enter the bloodstream. He goes on to say that the reaction and symptoms (including acne, sore throat, gas, bloating, and aching joints) can be instantaneous or occur even days later making it hard to distinguish which foods caused the reaction in the first place. Dr. Kellman also points out that this inflammatory reaction results in an outpouring of *insulin* into the system making weight loss (among other things) near impossible.[63] A wonderful side effect of removing these foods is that our immune system stops making the antibodies against them, and subsequently we begin to crave them less and less!

The crux of this matter is that of the health practitioners with a heavy focus on the gut, almost all of them recommend cutting out dairy. I agree with that recommendation and include it in the Gut Healing Protocol, however I allow some room for dairy on the Gut Nourishing Diet if you are able to tolerate and enjoy it.

What if I have access to raw, fermented dairy? For the duration of this protocol I recommend cutting out all dairy to reduce any chance of inflammation, then after following a slow reintroduction of dairy back into the diet (and a monitoring of its effects), you may include it on a regular basis should your newly-healed gut allow it.

Goat and sheep's milk are not encouraged for the time on this protocol and should be reintroduced slowly following the introduction principles explained in Chapter 8.

Ghee, which is clarified butter, may be used on the protocol on a regular basis as it does not contain the potentially inflammatory molecules in milk such as lactose or casein. It also contains around 25% highly anti-inflammatory short chain fatty acids.

The next obvious question is where do I get my calcium? I don't want osteoporosis! As Phillip Day points out in *Health Wars,* the countries with the highest rates of osteoporosis also tend to have the highest rates of dairy consumption, so let's not necessarily link dairy consumption with bone health *just because it contains calcium.*[64] The bone matrix is made up of numerous other substances such as boron, silica, zinc, and manganese and also relies on adequate levels of vitamin K (dependent predominantly on a healthy microbiome), vitamin D, and exercise! Rest assured there's more than dairy in the bone-health equation.

There is plenty of calcium, in bioavailable forms, in plant foods such as broccoli, spinach, and almonds and also in animal foods like sardines. One must also ask the question—*where does the cow get its calcium?* Added to this argument is the fact that by rebalancing our microbiome with beneficial microbes/bacteria we absorb calcium from our food more efficiently. There are theories that the beneficial bacteria in our guts can *biologically transmutate* other elements like silica into calcium.[65]

Sugar

I'm sure that in today's day and age I do not need to spend too much time elaborating on the detrimental effects that processed, and even some natural forms of sugar, have on our health, but put shortly, sugar may do the following:

- cause blood sugar imbalance

- increase the risk for diabetes, obesity, and heart disease

- suppress the immune system

- cause systemic mineral deficiencies

- accelerate aging

- damage DNA

- cause tooth decay

- cause inflammation of the brain

- increase stress and cause abnormal changes in behavior and mood

- massively disrupt the balance of the microbiome.[66]

In *That Sugar Film,* actor Damon Gameau embarks on a journey of self-experimentation, consuming foods commonly seen as "healthy" and often endorsed with "healthy stars" by dietary associations. He eats plenty of cereal, low-fat yogurt, muesli bars, and fruit juice and the results (without wanting to ruin the film) are astonishing. Throughout the film we see his health decline, his weight increase, and his overall vitality diminish. This is one story among many of how seemingly healthy foods actually contain significant amounts of hidden sugar, which has a hugely detrimental effect on health.

Dr. Weston A. Price in his book *Nutrition and Physical Degeneration,* describes in detail his journeys around the world to study the effects of sugar, flour, processed dairy, and table salt on different populations. He showed the significant decline in health (particularly dental and structural health) that cultures experienced when these foods were introduced into the diet. Notably, he showed that when these foods were removed, the subjects' health once again improved.[67]

We can ascertain quite clearly that refined sugar, whether hidden in low-fat foods, added to soft drinks, or even consumed in the form of refined white flour, is not a healthy food at all.

What about the natural sugars in fruit and some vegetables?

Here's where things get a little gray, because certainly fruits aren't *unhealthy*, as they provide antioxidants and fiber. It is true *however, that the majority of fruit is not recommended for the time you spend on the Gut Healing Protocol.* To explain the reason why, we need to go back to the womb. When a baby is born, he or she tumbles down the birth canal and is inoculated with loads of wonderful health-promoting bacteria. The majority of these bacteria thrive off natural sugars (prebiotics), while others might prefer proteins or fats. Mom's milk, by the second or third week, will actually be very sweet at this point and gives the healthy microbes sugar to feed on! When little baby finally begins solid foods and starts eating perhaps some banana and stewed apple, those naturally occurring sugars will also feed the beneficial bacteria inside his or her digestive tract. Now, if the *beneficial* bacteria are reduced or not present because for instance, the baby was born via C-section, fed formula, or given antibiotics, then what does the ingested sugar feed? Unfortunately, it often feeds the "bad" bugs.

Candida albicans is one particular species of yeast that is very quick to take control of the microbiome when excess sugar is available. Candida is normally a beneficial bowel yeast which feeds off excess sugars and heavy metals, however when there are not enough good bacteria present to control its growth, and when there is a frequent supply of sugar—*even from natural forms*--it can grow out of balance. Do not underestimate the power of this one species of yeast, as its health consequences can be dire, including organ failure, cancer, and death. Dr. Tullio Simoncini has written extensively on the cancer-fungal link and has actually had significant results injecting tumors with baking soda (or bicarbonate of soda—a strong alkalizing salt). Dr. Simoncini's work emphasizes the need for us to adopt an alkaline lifestyle if we are interested in preventing this disease.[68]

So, is an apple an apple regardless of the person consuming it? No, it isn't. This is why throughout our GHP journey the majority of fruits are not recommended—reintroducing these wonderful foods down the road, once we have established a beautiful inner ecosystem with lots of healthy bacteria, is a fantastic way to *truly* enjoy them and experience their health benefits.

On a gut-*nourishing* diet, fruit can be eaten in appropriate amounts. By sticking to low-sugar fruits like berries and apples, one can still manage their blood sugar quite effectively. Naturopath and nutritionist Kasey Willson recommends no more than 2-3 servings of fruit per day, however fruit like tomatoes, avocados, lemon, limes, and cucumbers can be eaten liberally. If you find yourself suffering from blood sugar fluctuations, try *only* consuming your carbohydrates (like fruit) 30 minutes before or after exercise.

What about sweet vegetables?

There are vegetables that we can indeed consume on the GHP even though they naturally contain some natural sugars. Carrots, beets, bell peppers, and sweet potatoes, all *in whole form* (not juiced), are encouraged on the protocol in moderate amounts due to their health-promoting and prebiotic properties.

It is important that we provide our microbes with enough fibers to feed upon, otherwise their presence in our digestive tract will only be transient!

Autoimmune Conditions

Those with autoimmune conditions such as multiple sclerosis, rheumatoid arthritis, or Hashimoto's may need to further restrict their diet in order to heal. In my experience working with clients and speaking with health practitioners, these patients need to take a somewhat firm approach to their gut-healing journey. Sufferers may benefit from excluding all nightshade vegetables and strictly limiting or avoiding altogether the intake of nuts and seeds. Being diligent about eating bone broth every day and taking gut supportive supplements is a necessity. Adding green tea and turmeric to the diet may also be beneficial, as these foods have been shown to reduce autoimmune reactions.[69]

If you do suffer from an autoimmune condition, consult your naturopath or integrative GP to determine the best approach for your unique body. Certainly, a good gut-healing diet, as outlined in this book with the aforementioned considerations, will help you on your healing journey.

Alcohol

Alcohol is clearly known for its "social" properties, but it is actually a carbohydrate. While on this protocol, it is highly recommended that you do not drink any alcoholic drinks, as doing so disrupts your microbiome and causes inflammation of the intestinal lining. Alcohol can actually multiply the number of gas-producing bacteria by a factor of up to a thousand![70] When you do finish the protocol and want to enjoy some social drinks, first stay clear of anything with added sugar, and try to stick with high-quality (often high-priced) spirits like vodka or tequila. Some organic red wine may also be okay.

If you're going out for dinner and don't want to miss out on some bubbles, try having some sparkling mineral water with fresh lemon squeezed in.

Artificial Sweeteners

We are going sugar-free on this protocol, but that doesn't mean the answers for all your sweet cravings lie with artificial sweeteners.

Artificial sweeteners such as aspartame, sucralose, and saccharin have been surrounded with controversy since their introduction into western diets. In fact, countless reports exist of their adverse effects on health. Complaints regarding blurred vision, headaches, and dizziness are common and other health ailments linked to the consumption of some artificial sweeteners include cancer, depression, moodiness, and weight gain.[71]

Most importantly, artificial sweeteners have a negative impact on our gut microbes. In a powerful study conducted by Israeli researchers, mice were fed a daily dose either of aspartame, sucralose, or saccharin, compared with another group receiving glucose or sucrose. After 11 weeks, the group receiving the artificial sweeteners showed abnormally high blood sugar levels *due to significant changes in the microbiome.* The researchers showed that after the time period, the artificial sweeteners seemed to create an "obese microbiome" whereby health issues like poor blood sugar regulation, diabetes, heart disease, and weight gain are more common. After being treated with an antibiotic, which presumably wiped out the "obese microbes," the mice seemed to return back to normal.[72]

Stevia seems to be a safe alternative as a low-calorie, sugar-free sweetener, however proceed with caution as some products contain not-so-healthy additives like sugar alcohols (erythritol, for instance, which can cause digestive complaints).

This throws into perspective the very idea of whether we need to have so much "sweetness" in our diets anyway. Once you've been on the Gut Healing Protocol for a while, you'll find that you can enjoy the sweetness in carrots, beets, and onions, as opposed to finding it only in chocolates and ice cream! One of the principles behind the GHP is to lose the taste for sweet or rather, to sensitize yourself to it so that you don't require massive doses of sweet foods to feel satisfied. Having an almond milk or having some pea or rice protein with stevia will not break the bank, but remember that we are trying to focus on real, whole foods during the program.

A common form of feedback I hear from those who undergo the Gut Healing Protocol is that they didn't realize how addicted they were to sweet foods! Participants had been "glancing over" their apple in the morning, their bliss ball after lunch, and their sneaky chocolate before bed! Although these foods can be acceptable in small-moderate amounts over the long-term, they can also feed an infection of pathogenic microbes, which is why it is important to cut them out while you rebalance your gut! After 8 to12 weeks on the program, these sneaky little addictions are quite easily managed.

Gut Nourishing Diets vs. the Gut Healing Protocol

As mentioned previously, a gut-*nourishing* diet is something you can adhere to for life. It is a relatively non-restrictive, whole food, and long-term approach to the maintenance of a healthy microbiome! If you have no digestive complaints, are not suffering from autoimmune disease, and feel like your gut is in a good place, then this may be a perfect type of diet for you to undertake.

The main difference between a simple gut-*nourishing* diet and a gut-*healing* diet is the intake of sugars and potentially inflammatory foods. On a gut-nourishing diet, one may consume plenty of whole food fibers from vegetables and fruits, eat healthy amounts of all nuts and seeds, and generally fare well on a diet encompassing most food groups. This is because, presumably, those without any digestive or health ailments have a strong, healthy microbiome to begin with which allows them to fully digest and then eliminate those foods.

With a healthy, diverse microbiome, one can eat a banana and actually thrive off the resistant starch found in the fruit because it feeds their gut microbes! Someone with a health condition related to the gut, however, may not benefit from eating a banana because they do not have the correct balance of microbes in place to deal with the sugar found in the fruit! They may have an overgrowth of candida, for instance (which may feed off the naturally occurring sugars in the banana), but not enough *probiotics* in the system to suppress the candida.

This may also relate to FODMAPs (Fermentable Oligosaccharides, Disaccharides, Monosaccharides And Polyols), which are a type of carbohydrate known to cause irritation in some people. FODMAP-containing foods are things like garlic, onion, and bread. Many people have been prescribed a FODMAP diet that eliminates certain carbohydrates that can cause an inflammatory response in their gut. This diet, although very effective at reducing symptoms, is still a symptom-based intervention, which doesn't necessarily address the underlying cause of such issues, namely the levels of inflammation within the gut.[73]

On a gut-nourishing diet, the regular intake of prebiotic fibers (including some FODMAPs) is heavily encouraged! Foods such as onions, garlic, beets, asparagus, chickpeas, legumes (in moderation and properly prepared), leeks, cashews, sweet potato, bananas, blackberries, tomatoes, and more should all be consumed with gusto as long as you feel you digest and eliminate them well! All these foods have been shown to provide fuel for your good gut bugs to thrive, and it is very important that you continually consume them.

Nuts and seeds will also fall in this category. Autoimmune conditions *can be* negatively impacted by the intake of too many nuts and seeds, so on a gut-healing program, these will need to be strictly controlled or eliminated altogether (at the discretion of the individual and/or their practitioner). On a gut-nourishing diet, one may sensibly consume up to a handful of nuts and seeds one to three times per day.

For those who feel like they need to be on a gut-healing protocol, some of these foods may cause unwanted symptoms such as bloating, autoimmune flare-ups and more. This is why it is important to regularly assess your health status to determine your specific gut health needs! There is no reason why, if you go through an effective gut-healing program, you shouldn't be able to consume the aforementioned foods once you rebalance your microbiome!

An apple is not an apple, nor are legumes, legumes; it depends on who is eating what and the state of their microbiome!

Over time, I have transitioned slowly onto a more flexible, gut-nourishing diet. With a greater appreciation for the role of variety and prebiotic fibers, I believe that once you put in the hard work in establishing microbiome health, this type of diet is an absolute winner.

Principles to carry over from a gut-*healing* protocol to a gut-*nourishing* diet include regular bone broth intake, moderate intake of sweet foods (and only whole-food varieties), regular probiotic supplementation, cyclic colostrum/Aloe vera supplementation, avoiding antibiotic use unless *absolutely necessary*, eating mindfully, and adhering to food-combining principles. (I go into depth about transitioning from gut healing to gut nourishing in Chapter 8.)

As always, the decision to transition onto the Gut Nourishing Diet should be made by you and your practitioner. As a general rule of thumb, you want to be free of any negative health symptoms for at least two to three months before relaxing the diet a little.

Now, let's look at the specifics of the Gut Healing Protocol.

All foods listed must also pass your inner nutritionist's approval—if you do not tolerate a food on the program, then do not force yourself to eat it! These lists are not all-encompassing, which is why it is important for you to understand the principles behind the GHP!

YES on the GHP Food List

VEGETABLES AND FRUIT

any green leafy vegetables & herbs	cauliflower
asparagus	celery
avocados	cucumbers
beets	garlic
red bell peppers	kale
broccoli	lemon/lime
Brussels sprouts	onions
butternut squash	spinach
cabbage	sweet potatoes
carrots	tomatoes

MEAT, FISH, AND EGGS (PREFERABLY ORGANIC, GRASS-FED, WILD-CAUGHT, OR PASTURED)

beef	eggs
bone broth	fresh fish
canned tuna/sardines/mackerel, occasionally if desired	lamb
	organ meats
chicken	

ALTERNATIVE PROTEIN

biofermented rice protein

pea protein

tempeh

NUTS AND SEEDS *1–2 small handfuls <u>per day</u>*

almonds

Brazil nuts (3-4 per day)

chia seeds (soaked best)

flax seeds (soaked best)

macadamia nuts

pumpkin seeds

walnuts

OILS

avocado oil

coconut cream (in small amounts)

coconut oil

ghee (from grass-fed, organic source)

macadamia oil

olive oil

SPICES/HERBS/CONDIMENTS

dulse flakes

fresh ginger

Great Lakes Gelatin

nori

pure organic stevia
(not erythritol—a sugar alcohol)

BEVERAGES

almond milk (unsweetened)

green/white/herbal teas

NO on the GHP Food List

VEGETABLES/BEANS

beans	mushrooms
chickpeas	pumpkin (butternut squash is permitted)
corn	snow peas
eggplant	turnips
maca	white potatoes
lentils	

GRAINS OR GRAIN ALTERNATIVES

amaranth	pasta/bread/wheat products/processed
buckwheat	and refined foods
quinoa	

MEAT

goat/sheep products

FERMENTED STAPLES

apple cider vinegar or fermented foods

miso

NUTS AND SEEDS

cashews	sesame seeds
chestnuts	sunflower seeds
hazelnuts	tahini
pine nuts	

BEVERAGES

black tea	coconut water

The 8 Week GHP — At a Glance

You determine portion sizes.

Chew thoroughly and slowly.

Eat until you are 80% full.

Don't count calories, count nutrients.

Eat in a relaxed, joyful state.

Eat 2 to 4 healthy meals per day, when you are hungry.

Be prepared.

Enjoy the process.

Take five deep diaphragmic breaths before your meals.

Eat an alkalizing, wholesome, real-food diet.

Embrace healthy fats.

Animal protein is a condiment—eat sensible portions.

*Enjoy bone broth on both the gut-healing
and gut-nourishing diets.*

Dietary Principals for the GHP

THE "IDEAL" PLATE

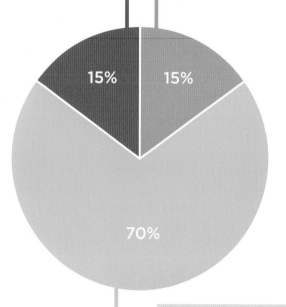

sweet vegetables
Sweet potatoes, butternut squash, carrots, and beets can be used here as healthy prebiotic additions to your meal!

protein & fat
Clean sources of animal protein and fat can go here, or plant-based sources like avocado or pesto!

low-sugar vegetables
Green leafy vegetables like celery and kale can go here alongside herbs, cucumbers, tomatoes, radishes, and capsicum/bell peppers!

something extra
Allow yourself some flexibility with these ratios. There may be some days where you feel you need more or less animal protein, or feel like a whole cooked meal like a curry or soup. Trust your body and enjoy each meal!

The Details

As we aim to alkalize the body, reduce inflammation, and heal the gut the majority of our plate should include colorful vegetables. If we can ensure that 70 to 80% of our meals consist of colorful, low-sugar vegetables the majority of the time, then we are well on our way to healing the gut. The remainder of the plate can include a palm-sized amount of sweeter vegetables like carrot, beet, sweet potato, or butternut squash, alongside a palm-sized amount of healthy protein and fat coming from animal or plant sources, depending on your preferences. Some good examples of healthy proteins and fat include roast lamb, olive oil or an olive oil-based dressing, avocado, and almond/basil pesto.

The Gut Healing Protocol in this book is an alkalizing, anti-inflammatory, anti-fungal, healing diet designed to help you move into a state where your innate healing power is activated. It embraces the power of fresh vegetables, herbs, and some low-sugar fruits, and we harness the grounding, nourishing properties of clean animal foods to create this healing environment.

One of the most common things people say when they enter this program is how easy and friendly it looks. Covering all the macronutrients and micronutrients (as much as possible), sweeping the system clean with plenty of healthy fiber, and eating a mindful, low-inflammatory diet are important principles of the GHP. This is not a complicated diet by any means. but it is important to avoid the foods not recommended on the program. as doing so will fully allow your healing power to re-establish.

One of the primary reasons we recommend such a significant quantity of vegetables in the program is because vegetables are a great source of fiber and is of extreme importance when establishing the health of the gut. During the Paleolithic era and in more recent generations, it may have been that people consumed more meat than vegetables and still thrived. It is my belief that in today's society, with our lack of movement, increased exposure to chemicals, use of oral medications, exposure to radiation, and dietary trends that disrupt the microbiome, we have an increased need for fiber to assist in cleansing our bodies. The benefits of fiber and subsequent digestion of fiber by the good bacteria in your gut has been extensively researched, and it is on the basis of this research (and some good old common sense) that we include such a high quantity of vegetables in this program.[74]

I find that starting off the day by making a large, colorful salad (like my Rainbow Salad from the recipes section on page 183) that can last over 2 to 3 meals helps keep you on track and will take the stress out of coming up with new foods to eat. Having a large salad as the "main" part of your meals while adding small condiments at different times makes decision-making easy.

You can rotate your condiment foods such as sardines, tuna, avocado, almond pesto, cauliflower fritters, or grilled chicken for variety, but maintain efficiency by using the same salad. Utilizing leftovers for breakfast will also take the stress out of cooking. Simply increase the quantity of ingredients when making dinner and have the leftovers for breakfast or lunch the next day.

With such a large intake of fiber, expect changes in your bowel movements. Over time, these should normalize to be regular, non-hazardous experiences. If you find that your digestion struggles with such a large amount of fiber you may need to drop back on the quantity you are eating and see how it goes. If you don't see improvements, consult with your practitioner about tailoring a more specific diet for you. It may be that you need to focus on lightly steamed or fried vegetables and lots of bone broth soups until you regain your digestive fire. Dr. Natasha Campbell-McBride recommends eating the soft meats from your bone broth as a starting point for those who need to rebuild their digestion. Once you feel like your digestion is back online, slowly reintroduce raw foods back into your diet at a rate that works for you, all the while monitoring your response.

Variety

It is of extreme importance that you consume a wide-variety of foods.

> *"15,000 years ago, our ancestors regularly ingested around 150 ingredients in a week. Most people nowadays consume fewer than twenty separate food items and many, if not most, of these are artificially refined."*[75]
>
> *—Dr. Tim Spector*

Consuming a wide variety of foods will ensure you do not develop allergies to foods and that you cover your micronutrient needs as much as possible. Some people get thrown off when they think they have to consume over 150 different foods per week, but we can aim for a much lower number and still be healthy. Don't put too much pressure on yourself, but try to include new herbs and spices into your cooking by creating an incredibly abundant spice cupboard. Try new varieties of animal protein, too. Rotating your animal protein on a daily basis is a fantastic idea and will prevent boredom—try different types of fish and land mammals and even try different types of eggs! All these small decisions will add points to your health balance.

Alkalinity

Dr. Robert O'Young has done tremendous work over the last 30 years researching the effects of food on blood pH levels and overall health. Dr. O'Young advises that the blood must maintain a slightly alkaline state of 7.34pH. In order to do this without drawing essential minerals from our bones, we need to eat an alkalizing diet.[76] Think about the blood system as a river that winds its way around your body delivering valuable nutrients to every single cell—if you have a polluted river you're going to have a polluted body! For reference here, I'll show you my blood under the microscope compared to someone else's blood (my Dad's—used with permission—sort of).

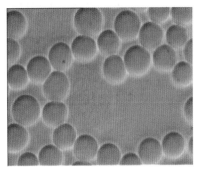
My blood

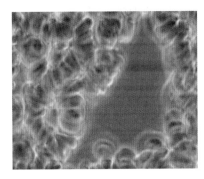
Dad's blood

It doesn't take a college degree to work out which blood would be more efficient at delivering nutrition to the cells does it? And yet it is an extremely common occurrence for people to have this sort of blood running around their body day in, day out, only to wonder why they feel tired and sluggish! A fantastic way for you to achieve healthier blood *immediately* is to earth/ground yourself; that is, get in contact with the earth's surface by walking barefoot on the sand, dirt, or grass, swimming in the ocean, or using an earthing sheet to sleep on or a mat to rest your feet on. Long term, dietary intervention will result in beautiful looking blood.

In this protocol, it is recommended that 80% of the food you consume should be alkalizing and 20% should be acidic to maintain a healthy balance between the two. Consuming some acidic foods like animal protein will help you stay emotionally grounded, too. A common misconception is that foods such as lemon and lime are acidic, when in fact their potassium bicarbonate levels exceed their citric acid levels, making them alkaline.

Exemplifying the miraculous power of using alkaline substances to heal the body is the work of Dr. Tullio Simoncini, an oncologist practicing from Rome, Italy. Dr. Simoncini regularly treats cancer tumors with the injection of sodium bicarbonate and has many successful patient recovery stories. According to Dr. Simoncicini, if we are interested in preventing cancer then we must overcome any infections of *Candida*.

> *"The Candida fungus is always found in cancer patients.*
> *This type of fungus is found in about 97% to 98% of cases.*
> *All research points to the presence of the Candida fungus.*
> *What matters is the correct interpretation."*[77]

According to Rice University, candida affects 70% of all people and is an adaptive, opportunistic organism that can easily become pathogenic.[78]

It can easily penetrate epithelial barriers, which means it can cross your intestinal lining and even your blood-brain barrier! Julia Koehler, Harvard University fellow in infectious disease, says that Candida is the predominant fungal infection behind human disease, claiming it is responsible for 60% of fungal infections acquired in hospitals and even killing 1 in 3 who have a systemic infection![79]

Donna Gates, founder of the Body Ecology Diet, writes of the potential symptoms of a Candida infection:

Bad breath

Bloating, belching, intestinal gas or pain

Constipation/diarrhea

Endometriosis or infertility

Fatigue

Impotence

Insomnia

Loss of sexual desire

Mood instability

Muscle aches

Pain or swelling of the joints

Poor memory and foggy thinking

Vaginal itching, burning, or discharge[80]

These symptoms are often associated with other diseases, making Candida tricky to diagnose as being a causal factor. Your digestive health and your attachment to sugary foods are key indicators to identify a Candida infection.

Remember that Candida is normally a beneficial bowel yeast, chewing up excess sugars and removing heavy metals from the body. It is only when there is an abundance of sugar and waste in your system *and* an absence of probiotic microbes that it can overpopulate the microbiome.

Remember that Candida is normally a beneficial bowel yeast, chewing up excess sugars and removing heavy metals from the body. It is only when there is an abundance of sugar and waste in your system *and* an absence of probiotic microbes that it can overpopulate the microbiome.

Importantly, an acidic environment is required for Candida to flourish and grow, so if we are to overcome this fungal overgrowth we must create an alkaline body which is done through eating a predominantly alkalizing diet.

Unfortunately, an overgrowth of Candida almost always results in *leaky gut* as the candida organisms burrow into the intestinal wall. Using anti-fungal herbs and supplements (explained further in the coming pages) is a great way to remove these deep-seeded infections.

Vegetarianism/Veganism and Gut Healing

If you are a vegetarian and participating in this protocol it can still work! You will be able to cover your nutritional needs as long as you are comfortable with at least having eggs, maybe fish, and some bone broth. It can be quite challenging as a vegetarian or vegan to effectively heal the gut, simply because many animal foods contribute to its proper healing. *Maintenance* of a healthy gut can indeed be possible on a vegetarian (and even vegan) diet if an emphasis is placed on whole foods from vegetables, fruits, nuts, and seeds. There is no shortage of fiber to feed healthy gut bugs from this type of diet.

One of the primary concerns about trying to improve gut health on vegetarian and vegan diets, though, is that when one excludes animal protein, often the macronutrient that takes its place is carbohydrate. This presents no major problem *unless* those carbohydrates come in processed, unhealthy forms like wheat and sugar, which is quite often the case with conventional eaters.

Simply by missing out on bone broth and colostrum, healing the gut can be quite difficult, but animal foods also offer another important benefit: blood sugar balance. Without adequate blood sugar balance, it is almost impossible to not crave sweet foods throughout the day, and adhering to the dietary guidelines in the GHP could be very difficult.

If you are a vegetarian and determined to attempt a gut-healing program, make sure you embrace the idea of healthy plant fats and proteins. By using nuts and seeds, avocados, plant oils, and more, you may be able to effectively nourish and ground yourself throughout the protocol. By supplementing with Aloe vera and/or slippery elm powder, you may be able to heal the gut lining as well.

Mushrooms and Nightshades

From some of the initial feedback I received about the foods to avoid in the Gut Health Protocol, it seemed like the end of the world. How would people survive without some of their favorite foods for 8-12 weeks?

The main reason we eliminate these foods in the GHP is because they can be potentially inflammatory within the gut, often without the consumer knowing! This may not be the case with everybody, however after working with practitioners and researching gut-related material, I have come to the conclusion that these foods are enough of an issue to list them as a "no." Tomatoes, although a nightshade (sometimes considered inflammatory), *are* encouraged on the protocol because they have specific *prebiotics* in them alongside some very powerful antioxidants, which outweighs any potential inflammatory effects. Capsicum (bell peppers) also fall into this category, *however* some people may still have negative reactions to it, so *listen to your body!*

Mushrooms are a fungus. When we are trying to control an environment that is most often "too fungated"—we need to reduce the foods we eat that may cause any potential flare-ups, and mushroom is one of them.

Many people will also go to war over the pumpkin issue. We have included *butternut* squash (which is in the same family) in the protocol, as it tends to have a lower glycemic index than other pumpkin varieties. Butternut squash offers an alternative to root vegetables like sweet potatoes, beets, and carrots for those who need it.

Once you have rebalanced your microbiome, these foods can be reintroduced into your diet as you like—so don't stress!

Animal Protein

Animal protein is a part of this protocol due to its strengthening, grounding and nourishing properties. Although animal protein is an integral part of this protocol, it is not a main dietary component. If taken in excess, animal protein may cause digestive stress and inflammation, so it is recommended in the program that *approximately* 20% of *most* of your meals come in the form of fats and proteins. This can be adjusted depending on your appetite and preferences—you do not have to eat animal protein at every meal, but it will be important in maintaining your blood sugar, keeping you satiated, and ensuring you are emotionally grounded throughout the protocol.

Cooking your animal protein is a good idea during this time to avoid the chances of any parasitic invaders entering the system. If raw fish is to be consumed, make sure that it has been frozen for 24 hours before being thawed or has been soaked in lemon juice for at least 12 hours (this works well for ceviche). Grilling or baking your animal protein is a great way to cook it as no oil is required. Gently frying animal protein is acceptable as well, but be sure about the quality of your oils—macadamia oil is fantastic, as it has a high smoke point, as does ghee, lard, grapeseed oil, and avocado oil. Coconut oil only has a smoke point of 350 degrees Fahrenheit (171 degrees C), so although I am still certainly an advocate for using coconut oil raw or for topical purposes, it may be best to avoid it for cooking. That being said, it may be that the medium-chain triglycerides in coconut oil are somehow protective at high temperatures. In tests done at De Montfort University by Professor Martin Grootveld, coconut oil was found to have the lowest levels of toxic aldehydes produced from cooking, while sunflower and corn oil produced the highest amounts.[81] I recommend you use stable oils to cook with *as much as possible* and cook at low to moderate temperatures as opposed to high temperature cooking. I strongly recommend against using a microwave oven to cook or reheat your food.

> *"I have lived temperately, eating little animal food... as a condiment for the vegetables which constitute my principal diet."*
> —Thomas Jefferson, US President

One of my favorite meals includes onion, sweet potato, and lamb chops. I simply cut the vegetables into small pieces and add them beside my chops on an oven tray, then I drizzle a little avocado oil (or sometimes olive oil) followed by some Himalayan salt and thyme, and throw them in the oven at 350 degrees Fahrenheit for 20 minutes. After cooking, I scrape it all onto a bed of salad greens for a perfect gut-nourishing meal that only requires about five minutes of actual prep time.

I also like poaching eggs. Doing so in water is fantastic, but in bone broth is even better because you get two meals at the end—the broth and the eggs. Slow cooking is safe and great for creating delicious recipes, but remember we want to eat most of our vegetables raw, so make the slow-cooked stuff only half the plate or less. As Dr. Damian Kristof says, that's food with a lot of fuel but not a lot of energy.

Ensure you enjoy good quality, healthy fats in your diet. They can make up to 80-90% of your *caloric* intake if you wish and can be sourced from things like avocado, almonds, walnuts, Brazil nuts, olive oil, macadamia oil, ghee, bone broth, and fatty cuts of meat, including the organs. Olive oil, it seems, has a very positive impact on the microbiome and as such it should be enjoyed liberally (ensure quality and organic sourcing). Tim Spector points out in *The Diet Myth* that 80% of the fatty acids and nutrients in olive oil reach the colon before full digestion. The microbes there feed on the fatty acids and polyphenols (antioxidant compounds), producing short-chain fatty acids, training our immune system, encouraging the growth of Lactobacillus bacteria and reducing the incidence of harmful, pathogenic microbes like E. coli. [82]

It is essential that you source your animal protein from reputable, safe farms that embrace organic/biodynamic farming practices. As Dr. Perlmutter points out, 80% of the antibiotics sold in the U.S. are used in livestock production! Those antibiotics don't simply disappear before we eat those same animals, so it is very important that the animal products you consume are not exposed to these chemicals. The organic industry is certainly not as good as it should be, but the fundamental principles it embraces should ensure your meat is free of harmful chemicals. I think one of the greatest and most affordable ways to source animal products is to get to know your butcher or farmer. Go and visit them, ask them about their farming principles, and develop a relationship with them. This also serves as a method for you to become connected with your food and community. Raising chickens is a fantastic way for you to harvest your own animal protein.

Food Combining

Throughout this protocol, you will naturally follow smart principles of food combining, but I want to explain this principle. Did you know that when you eat protein, it requires a highly **acidic** environment to be digested properly? The hydrochloric acid in your stomach, alongside powerful digestive enzymes like protease, break apart the protein you eat into small amino acids and peptide chains so that your small intestine can absorb them safely. What many people don't know is that starchy carbohydrates like those found in bread, pasta, rice and potatoes require an **alkaline** environment to be digested, and thus when proteins and starches are combined in a meal, they may result in a suboptimal digestive environment. This can result in the carbohydrates fermenting and producing gas, while the proteins begin to putrefy, toxifying the system.

When formulating your meals, on *and off* this program, it is recommended that you combine animal protein with non-starchy vegetables like salads (kale, spinach, lettuce) and optionally a small, palm-sized amount of starchy vegetables (carrot, beet, sweet potato). Having a sandwich, pasta dish, or rice curry with meat is not good food combining, nor is having that "raw treat" after your animal protein meal at dinner. Yes, down the line you may be able to break this rule from time to time on your more general gut-*nourishing* diet, but for the most part we should adhere to this principle.

When eating fats like almond basil pesto, avocado, or oily fish, it is important that you do not have an excessive amount of protein food at the same time, as excessive fats will slow down digestion leading to protein putrefaction. If you are having some lamb for instance with a big salad, it is permissible to add a small-to-moderate amount of fat like a salad dressing, avocado, or pesto, but anything excessive will slow digestion, so err on the side of caution.

When you exit this protocol and begin to include some sweeter fruits in the diet (like berries, apples, and pears), you should eat them alone on an empty stomach, preferably first thing in the morning.

Having excessive amounts of water with meals is also not ideal as this can lead to the dilution of digestive acids within the gut. It is recommended that you consume the majority of your water *between* meals and only *sip* during the meal. Wait at least 30 minutes after your meal before drinking any significant amounts of fluid.

One of the most common things I hear from people who adopt this principle is that their energy levels, especially in the morning, are increased dramatically. Sporting performance is often significantly improved as well.

Chewing

Who out there thoroughly chews their food? It's a question I ask that is quite often received with shifty, sideways looks around the room. Most people wolf down their food without savoring it. Mastication (the act of chewing) is an important step in preparing our food for digestion in the stomach.

I'll share with you a funny story. When I was young my family and I used to go out and catch squid. We came home one evening and cooked it all up, and yet it was too chewy for me. I didn't want to get told off, so I just swallowed around 12 squid rings whole. Later that evening I felt a little funny; about 45 minutes later I heaved up all 12 squid rings into the sink.

If we do not chew our food thoroughly in the mouth, this leads to improper digestion within the gut. Some experts say we should chew each mouthful around 30 times before we swallow—but who does that? Not many. Dr. Raphael Kellman teaches a great lesson in chewing by suggesting that you aim to be the last one finished at each meal—this will force you to slow down. Implementing some breathing exercises before meals will also serve to relax you so that you can be mindful about the food you are eating, which is particularly helpful when you eat by yourself.

Saying grace before a meal is a fantastic way to appreciate the food you're about to eat. This doesn't even have to be a religious habit, you can merely show thanks to the universe for delivering some awesome organic food to your table. Or, just show thanks to whoever cooked the meal! Gratitude has been shown to be one of the most beneficial emotions when it comes to overall health.

Chewing properly will also stimulate the cells within your teeth to maintain their density. This is why when we consume green smoothies, which are a great addition to any diet, I highly recommend you "chew" down the smoothie as opposed to just drinking it. Chewing will stimulate your teeth to become stronger, and it will stimulate the release of digestive fluids within the gut! Think about the foods you're eating, think about the energy that went into bringing them to your home, and finally think about the beautiful healing properties that they'll be passing on to you.

Eggs

Many detox or gut-healing programs do not include eggs in the diet. This is due to many people testing positive for antibodies to them. Eggs, though, are a super food and contain a plethora of nutrients such as vitamin D, acetylcholine, lecithin, and omega-3 fats, so why do people become allergic to them? First of all, it's extremely important to distinguish *caged* or *non-organic* eggs from organic, pasture-raised ones. The ratio of inflammatory chemicals in eggs is heavily reliant on what sort of food the laying hen had access to. For instance, the ratio of omega-6 fats (pro-inflammatory) to omega-3 fats (anti-inflammatory) is much higher in caged eggs, as opposed to those that are pasture-raised.[83] This alone can cause someone to react with inflammation after eating eggs even though they are not technically allergic to them. When consuming organic eggs people may not have any immune reaction at all.

If you are deeply concerned that eggs are a problem for you, I recommend you get a hair analysis allergy test done to determine exactly which foods "set off" your immune system. (Be sure to have them distinguish between organic and non-organic eggs, and also duck eggs.) If you sincerely feel like eggs are just not working for you, don't consume them. Otherwise, consume your eggs poached, sunny side up, or soft-boiled. The yolk should remain runny to ensure the high-quality fats and nutrients in it are still intact. Eggs should be balanced with green leafy vegetables like spinach or kale, and seasoned with some Himalayan or a good-quality sea salt.

Bio-Individuality

There is not one version of this diet that works best for everybody, as everyone has their own unique nutritional needs. We can only work within certain parameters to allow the gut to heal. For instance, if you feel like almonds (which are included on this protocol) disturb your gut and immune system, then it might be a good idea to remove them from your diet. If you do not have the budget for a hair analysis test to determine which exact foods you may be allergic to, you can always follow the age-old theory of seeing how you feel after you eat them.

The important point here is that *you* need to be the one to determine your perfect gut-supportive diet.

Carbohydrates

Many people are concerned that without 8 pounds of pasta per week they'll experience a dip in energy levels. First of all, there are plenty of healthy carbohydrates in the Gut Healing Protocol. Nature provides us with all manner of usable carbohydrates, such as carrots, beets, sweet potatoes, avocados, cucumbers, almonds, pumpkin seeds, and more, all of which are recommended on this program.

That being said, one of the positive effects of this protocol is that often participants shift into a state of mild *ketosis* which means instead of relying predominantly on sugar for cellular fuel, they begin to rely on fat! This is actually a very healthy state to be in because, as Dr. David Perlmutter puts it, fats (*ketones*) are a cleaner fuel with cascading health benefits.[84]

Ketones: Ketones are produced in the liver as a byproduct of fat metabolism when blood glucose and insulin levels are very low.

Ketosis: Ketosis is a condition in the body where ketones start to accumulate in the bloodstream to a point beyond which they can be utilized for energy.

Jimmy Moore describes ketosis wonderfully as "putting logs on the fire instead of twigs." Another fantastic benefit of being in ketosis is that people tend to lose that "emotional attachment" to food and quite often will forget to eat meals throughout the day—sounds pretty good, right? We also see a generalized decrease in inflammation throughout the body and some very positive impact on the brain from being in ketosis.

A ketogenic diet appears to be extremely beneficial for a variety of conditions from cancer, neurological disorders, diabetes, and epilepsy.[85][86] It's just like upgrading to a new, more fuel-efficient body.

Why fill your body up every 3 hours when you can fill it up only once or twice per day?

Interestingly, babies are actually born in ketosis, indicating it is a healthy, natural state. Being in ketosis or being more "fat-adapted" also has advantages for athletes as this helps them to avoid "hitting the wall" by optimizing fat-burning potential.[87]

Don't confuse ketosis with *ketoacidosis*. Ketosis is very natural and healthy. Ketoacidosis is a potentially life-threatening condition experienced by diabetics where blood sugar and blood ketone levels are high—normally these transverse and are never seen at high levels simultaneously.

> Why fill your body up every
> 3 hours when you can fill it up only once
> or twice per day?

Athletes may require more carbohydrates than the average person, as they need to constantly replace the muscle glycogen they regularly burn up with moderate- to high-intensity exercise. Those GHP participants who exercise at an intense rate (above 80% of maximum heart rate) more than three times per week can safely increase their carbohydrate intake by 10 to 15 percent.

Bone Broth

The addition of bone broth into the protocol is a necessity—you should have at least one serving per day while on the GHP. Bone broth, or just plain old stock, is a slow-cooked liquid that you make by simmering organic bones for 18 to 36 hours. Slow cooked broth releases valuable nutrition from the bones which can, among other things, work on healing the gut lining. In the bones and cartilage of animals lies a startlingly healing nutrient called *gelatin* and it seems that gelatin has the ability to reinforce the resistance of the gut lining against stress and inflammation-induced permeability.

Gelatin's short peptides called glyprolines consist of the amino acids glycine and proline, and these nutrients not only protect the gut lining but are easily absorbed into the blood stream where they act on the central nervous system. Glycine, arginine, and proline are amino acids which are highly anti-inflammatory, and as such will have a positive influence on the gut. Bone broth also contains good levels of chondroitin sulphates, glucosamine, and other compounds which are fantastic for maintaining joint health.[88]

When selecting bones or carcasses to make your bone broth, make sure that you purchase from organic, pasture-raised sources. Toxins are often stored in the fat and bones of mammals, so if you are buying non-organic bones and using those to make your broth, you'll be liberating those toxins into your stock! If you are on a tight budget, then prioritize by buying organic bones. These are still relatively cheap and they go a long way in the kitchen.

One of my favorite stocks is done with lamb shanks because after 3 to 4 hours you can remove the delicious meat and put the bones back in for another 20 hours. You may also add vegetables and herbs like carrot tops, garlic, onions, kale, leeks, rosemary, basil, and more to your broth to help flavor it. I like to add ginger and turmeric for extra color and a little zing. Although apple cider vinegar is not recommended while on the protocol, you can use it in your broths for its solvent properties. When you've finished boiling your broth and have allowed it to cool, it may develop a layer of fat on top. Do not throw this fat away—it can be kept in the broth, or you can scrape it off and store it to cook with later.

In Chapter 7, I will give you loads of gut-friendly recipes where you can really get a big bang for your buck with each broth.

Antifungals and Antimicrobials

Antifungal and antimicrobial herbs are important at certain times to overcome gastro-intestinal infections. However, the premise of this program is not to "attack" invaders of the body, but to support the gut and immune system so that the bad bugs can't get a foothold in the first place.

If you are certain that you need some anti-fungal/anti-parasitic products to help you overcome a yeast or parasitic infection, you may want to try any of the following:

Oregano oil

Pau D'arco tea or *inner bark* extract

Cinnamon

Black walnut

Wormwood

Echinacea

Grapefruit seed extract

Aluminum-free bi-carbonate soda (Take one teaspoon in water before bed for GI infections.)

Garlic (allicin extract)

Ginger

Colostrum (recommended on this program in "supplements")

Or a combination formula of the above. You can ask your local health store or naturopath about obtaining these products, or check out kalebrock.com for more resources.

It is a good idea to rotate at least 2 or 3 of these products every couple of days to prevent the yeast and parasites from adapting to them.

Naturally, by consuming a low-sugar diet along with natural anti-fungal (but also nourishing) herbs like basil, oregano, and thyme you can rest assured we are being "anti-fungal" at the same time as supporting the body and looking after our good bacteria. Anti-fungals can be used effectively as long as care is taken to replace beneficial bacteria in the system and to **change the systemic environment to an alkaline, healthy state so that the "bad guys" don't come back.**

By consuming a diet that is high in prebiotics, fuel for the good bacteria, we are shifting our internal environment to one that supports the growth and development of a balanced, healthy microbiome, and subsequently we are nurturing a healthy intestinal lining.

Water

You are made up of around 70% water, so doesn't it make sense to drink the highest quality water possible? Every single chemical reaction, cell, muscle and organ in your body relies on water. **Staying hydrated can be one of the best ways to maintain health and wellbeing throughout your life and is essential if you are to expect any benefit from this program.**

It is extremely difficult to heal the body when it is dehydrated. When it comes to the stomach and digestive system, it is particularly relevant to stay hydrated because an adequate water supply lines the stomach and prevents any damage occurring from the secretion of hydrochloric acid.

How much water and when?

For this program, I evaluated the work of Dr. Batmanghelidj and formed recommendations based upon this research. In his monumental book, *Your Body's Many Cries for Water*, he outlines fundamental principles we should all know about water. Batmanghelidj suggests drinking 0.033L of water (33mls) per kg of body weight to attain optimal hydration.[89 90] This can also be calculated as half your body weight in ounces of water per day.

EXAMPLE: 100kg (220 lbs.) male requires 3.3L (approx. 14 cups) of water per day plus additional water for exercise.

EXAMPLE: 70kg (154 lbs.) female requires 2.3L (approx. 10 cups) of water per day plus additional water for exercise.

In this program, I suggest that you add a pinch of Himalayan or high-quality sea salt to your drinking water (not so much that you can taste it) to increase the total dissolved solids and subsequent absorption of the water (which will also prevent you from weeing all day).

Drinking 500-750mls (2 to 3 cups) of pure water as soon as you wake up is a fantastic way to rehydrate after your body hasn't had access to water all night. It is also one of the best ways to shed excess weight and toxins, because your body can relax knowing it has a constant supply of water. If you wish, you can do a glass of water with fresh lemon juice squeezed into it, but be sure to have a glass of fresh water afterwards to protect your teeth.

Where should I get my water?

There is a lot of controversy about the consumption of municipal waters that often contain fluoride and chlorine. This is not a topic that we will explore in-depth in this book. That being said, **chlorine and fluoride are strong antimicrobial substances**, which is why we use them to ensure a clean, uncontaminated water supply. However, due to these properties, chlorine and fluoride can indeed have a negative impact on your microbiome when you consume them! This is just common sense— not a philosophical standpoint. If we are interested in maintaining the balance of healthy bacteria within the GI tract, then we should not be ingesting water that has been treated with these chemicals.

So, what's the answer? Filtered water does have its advantages because it is relatively cheap and easy to obtain. Please note that if you are using something like a Reverse Osmosis filter, then it is imperative that you place a high-quality salt into *all your drinking water*, otherwise you may enter hyponatremia, a condition whereby your electrolytes become too diluted.

Water is a source of information for your body—it is nutrition. In the GHP we run on the principle that spring water should be sourced and consumed as your principle drinking water.[91] A way to make this convenient is to get your spring water delivered, as many companies offer this service now.

Smoothies and Juices

On this protocol, it is recommended that you have regular green smoothies. Green smoothies are a cool way to bring loads of nutrition into your body in an easy, quick, digestible way. Blending vegetables and low-sugar fruits in a high-quality blender in a sense predigests them, taking the burden off your digestive system, while still ensuring you receive the smoothie's nutrition.

Smoothies are great because they are quick and easy to make, so for the time-strapped parent or student they can be a healthy savior! It is recommended that when you drink your green smoothie, you actually *chew* it. By chewing your green smoothie on the way down, you're stimulating digestive fluids to flow into the stomach and also being more mindful of the food you consume.

Green smoothies are particularly helpful to keep you regular because the high fiber content will sweep the digestive system, making for some seriously awesome (and green) poo. For green smoothies on this protocol, use this template:

> 1 big handful greens of choice (kale, spinach, collards, lettuce, parsley)
>
> 1 lemon or lime
>
> 1 palm-sized serving of healthy fats (avocado, almonds, olive oil, soaked chia seeds)
>
> 1 to 2 cups (250-500mls) water
>
> Place all ingredients into a high-speed blender and blend until smooth!

Juice can also be a fantastic way for you to bring nutrition into the body in a highly concentrated form, however it is recommended that you have smoothies rather than juice on this protocol. This is because when you remove all the fiber from a food, you increase its glycemic load. That is, if you remove all the fiber from a carrot, you're left with a lot of sugar, and that sugar may cause insulin spikes, dampen the immune system, and most importantly may *feed unhealthy microbes within your gut!*

As mentioned previously, fiber is an extremely important part of the protocol as it sweeps the digestive system clean and provides nourishment for our friendly microbes. Remember those microbes produce awesome nutrients for us like butyric acid *only when there is good fiber* coming into the system. Green juices, for instance those made with kale, celery, cucumber, and a little lemon may be consumed on an irregular basis, but do not solely rely on them.

Coffee (Good News!)

Coffee has gotten a bad rap over the past few decades as being somewhat toxic to the human body, but this is quite far from the truth; at least that's what the science is now telling us.

The intake of coffee seems to be positively associated with a healthier microbiome[92] and may even reduce intestinal permeability.[93] In a study performed in Germany, researchers determined that coffee contains fiber which healthy microbes can digest readily, producing important nutritional byproducts for us. The researchers showed a 60% boost in numbers of the beneficial microbial species Bacteroides and Prevotella. Levels of short chain fatty acids such as acetic acid, propionic acid, and butyric acid were also increased; all beneficial to gut health.[94] Science has gone back and forth for a long time on the issue of coffee, but it seems there is certainly some benefit to drinking it. Another study performed in Finland showed that "moderate" coffee drinkers (between a whopping 3 and 5 cups per day) showed a 65% decreased risk for developing Alzheimer's disease.[95]

While on the GHP, have one coffee per day, no more. It is best to proceed with caution. Coffee *can* exacerbate a leaky gut, so it is important to follow a few guidelines when consuming it:

Don't add sugar or dairy milk to your coffee, although some stevia may be used.

Consume coffee within 20 minutes after a meal, not before.

Add some form of fat (coconut oil/ghee/unsweetened almond milk) to buffer the effects of the coffee on the gut and to slow the release of the caffeine into your system.

Choose only organic coffee, as coffee is one of the most heavily sprayed crops in the world.

Herbal teas such as tulsi, dandelion, and chamomile and green and white tea can be consumed on a regular basis, taking care that this does not replace your drinking water! Tulsi is a fantastic herbal tea that I love, as it has adaptogenic properties which support the adrenals, liver, and vital organs. Dandelion is delicious (roasted dandelion is a great replacement for coffee) and is a powerful liver tonic. Turmeric lattes have become increasingly popular and are a great drink to enjoy while on the GHP.

Oil Pulling

An effective way for you to ensure the health of your oral biome is by implementing some oil pulling into your regime. The importance of the oral biome has been highlighted throughout the last 80 years by dentists such as Dr. Weston A. Price. (Dr. Price is known for taking the tooth of a patient who had died of liver cancer, inserting it under the skin of a rabbit, and reporting that weeks later the rabbit died of liver cancer.[96]) He showed that the microbes that live in your mouth can have a significant impact on the entire body.

Oil pulling is an optional intervention that you can try during the gut health protocol, so let's delve into it.

Oil Pulling is an ancient Ayurvedic method whereby one swishes a plant-based oil around the mouth for 5 to 20 minutes, then spits the oil out into the trash or garden. (*Don't put it down the sink, or you'll clog your drains*). Coconut, sesame, or olive oil are often used, and the belief is that the solvent properties of these oils pull bacteria and toxins from the mouth and bloodstream (remember blood circulates readily in the tissues of the mouth and is subject to diffusion). There seems to be a significant benefit to oil pulling on oral health, and Ayurvedic practitioners recommend it for healing bleeding gums, tooth decay, cracked lips, and for strengthening the teeth, gums, and jaw.

From personal use, I have experienced great benefits from incorporating oil pulling into my regime. At one point, I had pain from wisdom teeth coming through. Every time I was in pain, I simply used one tablespoon of coconut oil and oil pulled for 10 to 15 minutes until the pain went away. I've also had trouble with my teeth over the years due to past eating behaviors, and oil pulling definitely helps keep them strong and healthy.

A 2009 study published in the Indian Journal of Dental Research found that pulling with sesame oil reduced plaque and lowered levels of pathogenic microorganisms in the plaque of adolescents with plaque-induced gingivitis.[97] There have been multiple studies to show that oil pulling is as effective as mouthwash at reducing bad breath.[98]

One of the key principles of oil pulling is that it reduces pathogenic microbial levels in the mouth which has a "flow on" effect throughout the body. If these toxins are allowed to enter the bloodstream, they can become a systemic problem; pulling them out of the mouth with oil prevents this occurring. Any good holistic dentist will tell you that each tooth is connected to a vital organ via meridian channels in the body and if you are experiencing the decay of a tooth on the heart channel for instance, it could be affecting the heart, too. This throws into perspective the shortcomings of modern dentistry whereby the teeth are often treated as being completely separate from the rest of the body.[99]

Here's how to pull oil:

> Take one tablespoon of organic, food-grade olive oil, coconut oil, or sesame oil and place it in your mouth.

> Calmly swish the oil and pull it through your teeth—taking care not to swallow any of the oil.

> After 5 to 15 minutes, spit out the oil into the garden or trash.

> Rinse your mouth with a non-toxic mouthwash or brush with fluoride-free toothpaste.

Oil pulling has a myriad of health benefits, so if you have the time and patience (it gets easier the more you do it), then I highly recommend you add it to your regimen.

Stress

Dr. Bruce Lipton, in his book *The Biology of Belief,* puts forth a stunning narration of the power of our thoughts and beliefs over the rest of our body. The power of your thoughts should not be understated, and people like Lipton suggest that we will never overcome illness if we are stressed. When stressed, the long-term activation of the HPA axis (hypothalamus, pituitary, and adrenals) and subsequent depletion of vitality is one thing, but negative changes can also occur at the cellular and DNA level which disrupt healing.[100]

Everybody gets stressed. This is just a normal part of living, and indeed it can be said that *some stress* can be healthy. Examples of good stress may be surfing a perfect wave that scares you, or getting excited after conducting a successful presentation at work, but it's when stress becomes chronic that we should be concerned.

Having even low-grade emotional stress is like trying to walk up a hill towing an anchor behind you; it hinders your efforts to get to the top and become healthy.

Having even low-grade emotional stress is like trying to walk up a hill towing an anchor behind you; it hinders your efforts to get to the top and become healthy.

You can reduce if not eliminate stress effectively with some breathing exercises. It is recommended in the protocol that you practice this breathing technique before each meal. As Paul Chek says, you need to *rest and digest.* If you're in a stressed-out state, energy reserves aren't flowing to your stomach for digestion, they are hanging out in your muscles waiting for that sabre-tooth to come and grab you! When we eat in a relaxed, calm state, we chew more thoroughly, we are mindful of the food we eat and we appreciate it more. We satiate easily and *actually digest the food more thoroughly,* drawing the life-giving nutrients we need. Bring this calm, relaxed state about by diaphragmatically breathing for five breaths before you eat.

Here's how to breathe diaphragmatically:

> Rest your hand on your belly button.

> Breathe in through your nose slowly, ensuring your belly expands outwards against your hand—this is your diaphragm expanding the chest cavity. Your chest should be the last thing to expand.

> Hold the breath for a few seconds then…

Breathe slowly out through your mouth or nose, which-ever feels right, until your belly feels like it cannot pull in any further.

Repeat the process for five breaths before each meal. This will bring you into a parasympathetic (rest and digest) state where your immune system is strong, your digestive fire is optimized and you can think more clearly. An added benefit to breathing this way is that it pumps the cerebral spinal fluid among the vertebrae, keeping your spine and nervous system well-nourished.[101]

Sleep

Adequate sleep quantity *and quality* are extremely important when it comes to healing your body from any illness. Sleep can be one of the most restorative practices that we have access to; if we get it right. One of the most common stories I hear from people who have illnesses is that they fall asleep on the couch watching TV, and then they wake up around midnight, turn off the TV, and go to bed. Firstly, this is det-rimental to your *mental* health because the (mostly) negative content from the TV filters straight into your unconscious mind. Secondly, this is harmful to your *physical* health because the light information from the TV actually reduces your ability to sleep *deeply*. Thirdly, you're often in an extremely poor posture when watching TV. and sleeping *in* that posture is certainly harmful to your spine and nervous system.

Sleep, according to the research has multiple restorative effects on the body including muscle growth, tissue repair, protein synthesis, and the release of growth hormone.[102] Sleep is so important that in studies, animals that are kept awake and not allowed to sleep lose all function of their immune system and die within weeks. Sleep's effects on the brain are well known by the layperson of course. Just try and go without a good night's sleep and you'll find yourself easily stressed, less able to deal with mental challenges, and subsequently *less able to stick to your dietary goals*. Inadequate sleep also drains your adrenal glands and may spike your cortisol to chronically high levels, resulting in numerous health challenges.[103] Adequate sleep allows the brain to maintain its plasticity, the ability to learn and remember things.

> Without a good night's sleep, you'll find yourself easily stressed, less able to deal with mental challenges, and subsequently less able to stick to your dietary goals.

Cultivate healthy sleep habits by mimicking natural sleeping situations. Create your own sleep sanctuary by ensuring you have a dark room to sleep in, turning off the Wi-Fi in your home as well as the electrical appliances in your room, setting your phone to airplane mode, and maintaining access to fresh air.

Vitamin D

On my podcast on iTunes, I interviewed Dr. John Cannell from the Vitamin D Council (of Australia), arguably the world's leading expert on the effects of Vitamin D on the human body. What I learned during this interview is that vitamin D *plays an essential role in maintaining optimal health and functioning*, especially of the immune system. Vitamin D actually up-regulates 10% of the human genome! This means that it has strong epigenetic powers ("above" genetics) which can have a large influence on the expression of different genes, triggering disease or vitality.[104] Daily sunlight also has a profound impact on the balance of our hormones and neurotransmitters because it acts as an external signal for our circadian rhythm. This point was supported in a 1998 experiment published in *Science* where researchers were able to wake sleeping subjects and balance their sleep/wake cycle by shining a light on the back of their knees.[105]

An important point when it comes to sun exposure is that it should be done *in the middle of the day when the sun is around its zenith.* This is almost blasphemy in Australia where skin cancers are extremely common. However, *ideal* sun exposure *should not lead to getting sunburned*, as this can be dangerous. The reason experts like Dr. John Cannell recommend getting sunshine in the middle of the day is because the ratios of beneficial UVB rays to damaging UVA rays are optimum, meaning we create the most vitamin D with least damage to the skin during this time. Dr. Cannell recommends staying in the sun about *half the time it takes you to go pink* to optimize your vitamin D levels and to use the rule of thumb that if your shadow is taller than you, then you are sunbathing at the wrong time of day and will not benefit by making enough vitamin D.[106]

Sunshine is also fantastic because it kills pathogenic microbes. We see this when a citrus fruit drops off a tree and ripens on the ground—it looks fantastic and healthy on the sun-exposed side, but when we pick it up, it's all moldy and gross on the underside. So, if you are interested in overcoming a fungal infection, improving your immune system, activating your genetic potential, and healing your gut, then it is important to optimize sun exposure.

If you have a regular 9-to-5 office job and are coming home feeling exhausted and *wi-fried*, then you should prioritize spending your lunch breaks outdoors. Get your bare feet on the earth in a nearby park if you can, and do some breathing exercises while you soak up the sun—you'll feel all the better for it and your afternoon productivity will skyrocket.

Exercise

Exercise is a fundamental part of being healthy. There are some who would say it is the most fundamental part of living a healthy life, and in some respects, I would certainly agree. I remember one time when I was traveling through Indonesia, I was on Nusa Lembongan, a beautiful little island just off Bali and my girlfriend and I went for a ride on a scooter. We rode up into the hills and got lost, bouncing our way through holes and ditches until we somehow ended up on a farm overlooking the beautiful sunset. It was so quiet except for the sniff and shuffle of chickens and cattle, but then we heard someone cackle. It was a cheeky, knowing laugh coming from above us; we looked up and saw a wrinkled but healthy man sitting in the tree above us. He had a long machete and was cutting off branches from the tree. We watched as he continued his job with incredible alacrity for someone so old (we estimated around 80 or 90). He bounced from tree to tree with his ladder and powered on throughout the sunset. He came down eventually and then sat there eating white rice out of a banana leaf.

I tell you this story because it threw into contrast for me the contradictions we have of diet and health around the world. This man looked extremely healthy and certainly moved as if he were, and yet here he was eating a plain, somewhat nutritionally-void bowl of rice, which he'd probably subsisted on throughout his life. Maybe he wasn't going to live to be 120, maybe he wasn't exactly thriving all the time (though he could have fooled me), but compared to 80- to 90-year-olds here in the West, this man was doing incredibly well. He obviously lived an active lifestyle which seems to be the common theme in the research on long-timers throughout the world.

"Exercise stimulates the immune system in beneficial ways, then the immune system in turn sends chemical signals to the microbes in our guts. But it could also work

the other way around, as exercise alone can also influence the gut microbiota composition directly."[107]

> —Dr. Tim Spector

The benefits of exercise are well known. It increases/maintains bone-density, increases/maintains muscle mass, improves insulin sensitivity, and there is now even research showing that it may improve the health of your microbiome![108] In a study performed on rats, where rats who ran 3.5km on a running wheel were tested against those who didn't run, twice the rate of the beneficial short-chain fatty acid butyrate (that's the GABA we spoke of earlier) was found in the running rats' guts compared to the non-runners. Research done by The American Gut Project has shown that the strongest factor found to date affecting the richness of one's microbiome is the amount of exercise they do.[109] Researchers at this time are unsure of the mechanisms by which exercise improves the microbiome; it could well be that people who exercise regularly are also interested in a healthy diet, which contributes to having healthier microbes.

I actually believe that it is the lactic acid produced during exercise that has a beneficial effect on the microbiome, as we have many health promoting bacteria like the *lactobacillus* family that love and produce lactic acid. Do you remember when you were young, exercising to the point where you wanted to throw up? That's actually your body telling you that lactic acid has moved into the stomach and is overloading it to the point of hitting the "eject" button. Obviously, this is not a healthy situation, but it is possible micro-doses of lactic acid being pumped from the working muscles and diffusing into the stomach may provide nourishment to our friendly microbes. We'll see if this theory holds true over time.

Another key benefit from exercise is that it pumps the lymphatic system. This toxin-holding system needs to be actively pumped by the heart through movement to release toxins and rid them from the system, hence the importance of *moving every day.*

The lymphatic system needs to be actively pumped by the heart through movement to release toxins and rid them from the system, hence the importance of *moving every day*.

Movement doesn't have to be strenuous every day. Although weight training, squatting, lifting, and lunging are all essential movement patterns, a long-term approach to exercise can be fun and enjoyable nonetheless. Make exercise incidental from doing something you enjoy. For me it's surfing. For you it might be walking the dog or walking with friends, playing soccer or football, or learning a new skill like yoga or gymnastics.

Exercise can be done in the bedroom by having sex with a partner. It is important to note that there is a constant exchange of microbes between sexual partners, so it is very important for you to encourage your *friend* to optimize their microbiome, too.

Exercise will have a profound impact on your health and wellness, so give your body the care it deserves by doing it every day.

The Window of Power

With the demands of everyday living upon us, it can be hard to implement new health strategies into our lives. One of the best ways you can "hit the nail on the head" is to combine many of these health interventions into a small-time window that you set aside every single day.

When I speak in the corporate world I call it your BEEMS or BEMS time.

BEEMS:

Breathe

Eat *(if you're hungry)*

Earth

Move

Sunshine

Setting aside at least 30 minutes per day (or even better 60 minutes) to go through your health activities: diaphragmatic breathing, eating healthy food (if you're hungry), earthing, moving, and getting some sunshine is a great way to be time efficient. It's also a good idea for you to increase your productivity in everyday life or work, as these activities ensure an adequate supply of energy to the brain, healthy blood flow, and hormonal health.

So perhaps your time for BEEMS is first thing in the morning. Can you get up and go for a barefoot walk on the beach coupled with deep breathing? If so, you're ticking off 4 of the above 5 points already. And then if you follow it up with a healthy breakfast, you're on your way to cultivating health and vitality in your life.

Your health outcomes are a reflection of the degree to which you cultivate wellness.

I cannot emphasize this enough. No one is going to be more responsible for your application of this, or any other, program than you. If you approach your gut healing with an 80/20 mindset, expect 80% of the results. If you approach it with a 100% mindset, then expect 100% of the results.

Although this is suggested as an 8-week protocol, I encourage you to think about this in a more long-term way. As I mentioned early on in the book, you're better off being 80% perfect for the rest of your life than 100% perfect for just 12 weeks. There are times when I am traveling the world and can only do the best that I can with what's available. For me, logic comes before rules, so don't make yourself crazy while outside your typical environment.

If you can commit to it, I strongly urge you to follow the program 100% while you're healing your gut, but also keep in mind that if any slip ups do occur, **it's not an excuse for you to fall off the wagon**; just accept it, move on, and be awesome tomorrow. A gut-nourishing diet can be followed in a much more relaxed manner, but if you're working hard to help your gut heal from past behaviors or interventions, then it is best to be strict.

However, using a dietary slip up as an excuse to completely throw away your gut-healing journey is the easy way out. The harder thing to do, and the right thing to do, is to get back on the train with positivity and acceptance. Don't dwell on past decisions, look forward and focus on how good you're going to be from now on.

We live in a world where the saying "everything in moderation" has become quite popular. I think it's popular because it gives people an "out" when they delve into some not-so-ideal behaviors like binge drinking for instance. Unfortunately, in most cases, the "moderation" often evolves from once per month to once per week, and from once per week to once per day. It's the same with food, one of the most common experiences people have on this protocol is that if they "slip up," it leads to a cascading decline in their participation rate in the rest of the program.

So, for at least 8 weeks of your life, be as good as you can when it comes to following the guidelines in this protocol; you'll find by the end of week number 2 or 3 it won't be as hard to stay on track anymore.

Why?

Why did you buy this book? Why did you start this protocol?

Initially you might say something like "I just want to lose weight," or "I just want to fix my digestion and acne."

And these would be fine answers. But what if you asked the follow-up question to "why?" with "Why do I want to fix my acne? Why do I want to lose weight?" Often it's these follow-up questions which point us to the real reason for our embarking on any health program. These questions also lead us to our "one thing" or "overarching dream" in life. Think about how a highly functioning healthy body might help you achieve your overarching dream? Might it make you a better mom or dad? Might it make you a better athlete or entrepreneur or CEO? The answer is almost always "yes" because most people can't achieve their overarching dream from the hospital bed or when they're sick and tired.

"He who has a why to live for can bear almost any how."
—Nietzsche

If you're sick and tired of being sick and tired, then now is the time to act. Pick a date, commit to it, create some accountability by telling people (social media is great for this; you can find awesome sharing tools at www.kalebrock.com.au/ghp), and enjoy the journey to your best self.

Tell your local health store or naturopath what you're doing for the next few months. Tell them you're on a gut-healing journey and allow them to give you encouragement and advice throughout. Having a supportive network will absolutely help you achieve your health goals.

CHAPTER 5

Supplementation

I must emphasize that this information cannot be used in place of medical advice. Speak with your integrative GP or favorite qualified wellness practitioner before taking any supplements. Visit kalebrock.com *for more info.*

Supplementation is going to be key in achieving the ideal results for you on this program. The GHP harnesses the power of science and technology in a way that assists the body to heal. One could rave on about how supplements are not natural and we can get everything we need from our diets, but that simply isn't true anymore. One must also consider that flying, being exposed to radiation and EMFs, our levels of stress, antibiotics, medications, processed food, and air pollution are not natural either, and if we are interested in balancing our toxic load, then it is certainly in our best interest to embrace the power of nutrient supplementation.

You *can* choose to continue on the protocol without supplementation, and chances are you'll still achieve good results. Incredible, fantastic results may be hard to achieve without added nutrition; here's why.

Eris Watkins, Australian naturopath, points out that children born 50-100 years ago were born into a world with a lot of nutrition and low amounts of toxicity. In modern times, it's the complete opposite: children are being born into a world with high amounts of toxicity and low amounts of nutrition. A study conducted by the Environmental Working Group found extremely worrying levels of toxicity among newborn infants:

"...researchers at two major laboratories found an average of 200 industrial chemicals and pollutants in umbilical cord blood from 10 babies born in August and September of 2004 in U.S. hospitals. Tests revealed a total of 287 chemicals in the group. The umbilical cord blood of these 10 children, collected by Red Cross after the cord was cut, harboured pesticides, consumer product ingredients, and wastes from burning coal, gasoline, and garbage."[110]

Many of us think it quite natural now to peruse the shopping aisles to gather our food, whereas this is actually a really unnatural concept. Due to modern living and socio-economic demands, we are no longer consuming food in season, meaning nutrient levels are out of balance. We're spraying heavily with pesticides and herbicides, storing fresh foods for up to 10 months at a time (reducing their nutritive value), and artificially ripening many fruits with substances like ethylene gas![111]

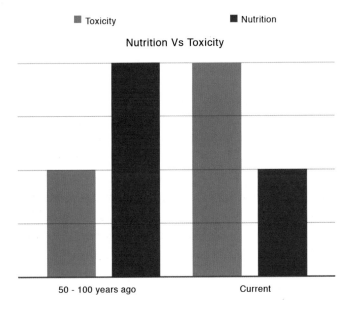

■ Toxicity   ■ Nutrition

Nutrition Vs Toxicity

50 - 100 years ago   Current

This is a big issue, and it's one that's being glanced over by mainstream and alternative outlets alike. If we are interested in attaining optimal health, then fresh, organic, homegrown food is the direction we have to head in when it comes to feeding the world's population.

Often, it is this discrepancy in overall nutrition that results in an imbalanced state. If you're going to bed every evening with so much toxicity to deal with yet only a small amount of nutrition, you can see why some people wake in the morning feeling as if they've been run over by a truck and need multiple cups of coffee before they can get going.

So, in a general sense we have a negative health balance, but we're also missing specific micronutrients that play a major role in our health. This is where supplementation can be used to "top up" the health bank balance so that we can begin to thrive again. You must remember our bodies are still living *biologically* in an era where all food was wild-harvested and full of bioavailable nutrition. In order for us to thrive, we need to honor our bodies' primordial needs.

Based on my research, following are the top gut-health supplements which I recommend you harness during your gut-healing program.

Probiotics

Using therapeutic, pharmaceutical-grade probiotic formulas is going to be key in healing your gut lining. As we've ascertained throughout this book so far, they're integral to maintaining gut integrity.

But let's talk about specific strains for a moment and go into why we may be better off, in the initial stages of our gut-healing program, to stick to probiotic *supplements* as opposed to probiotic *foods*.

You may recall the segmented filamentous bacteria that we spoke of previously. These are bacteria which are passed from Mom to you during the birthing process, and it is these bacteria that move into your GI tract and "set up shop." These initial seedlings of bacteria are integral in *training the immune system to accept such strains of bacteria as being friendly, beneficial, and native to the host.* These bacteria are the "mother" strains, if you will, and will form the default microbiome for young baby for the rest of his or her life.[112]

One thing we must point out is that babies are actually born with a leaky gut *by design.* This is to allow important nutrients in Mom's colostrum to move into the bloodstream immediately to fortify the immune system and set up growth trends. Once this process occurs, the gut is stimulated to seal, whereby a healthy mucous begins to develop around the gut lining; perfect "soil" for the "seeds" (bacteria) to adhere to. This sets up a happy, friendly environment for the good microbes who will inhabit the gut.

Because so many human beings now have increased intestinal permeability (a leaky gut), and it is probably one of the primary reasons for you to participate in this protocol, it is in our best interest to use strains of bacteria that were *most likely* present at birth and to mimic the segmented filamentous bacteria you were inoculated with. It is nearly impossible for us to determine exactly the bacterial species which you received from Mom at birth, but according to most prominent experts in the field of microbiology two species dominate: ***Lactobacillus and Bifidobacteria.***[113]

It is not by accident then that it is these two species of bacteria that are the most widely studied or that their benefits have been established as far-reaching. Bifidobacteria love breastmilk, for instance, and Lactobacillus bacteria ferment carbohydrates to form lactic acid which creates an environment conducive to their ongoing survival and growth. Scientists have been able to boost positive brain chemicals like brain-derived neurotrophic factor (BDNF) in mice just by inoculating them with Bifidobacteria.[114] Lactobacillus and Bifidobacteria seem to be species of bacteria that "work well" in the presence of a leaky gut and even can reduce the "leakiness" of the gut.[115] These bacteria inundate a newborn baby which, theoretically speaking, should cause an immune reaction, however this is not the case. Let's explain further.

A species of yeast that has been studied extensively is *Saccharomyces boulardii,* and although overall its effects seem to be very positive, some people have intolerances to it and may experience a negative skin rash or other reaction after taking it. A rash is a sign of immunological disturbance. Now, what else results in the breakout of a rash? Allergies and food intolerances. What process are we now attributing the cause of allergies and food intolerances to? *Increased intestinal permeability.* It is the leaky gut which allows certain species of bacteria or yeast—though beneficial within the gut, they are not elsewhere—into the bloodstream *where they are not recognized as being useful,* and as a result are met by an immune response. An immune response with collateral damage that we see as a red rash on the skin.

This is why in the GHP we encourage you to supplement with probiotic formulas which contain high numbers (in the trillions or high billions of CFUs is best) of Lactobacillus and Bifidobacteria (substrains included), as these are the same species of bacteria that you *most likely* received from Mom at birth and as such work best with your leaky gut condition. It is for this reason that we also encourage you to avoid fermented foods for the GHP, which contain a mixture of beneficial bacteria and yeast, until we have healed and sealed your gut lining. These foods can be very healthy for you, but in order to get the benefits from them that you should, your gut lining needs to have optimal integrity.

Probiotic supplements might include strains such as *Lactobacillus acidophilus, Lactobacillus plantarum,*[116] *Lactobacillus brevis, Bifidobacterium lactis*[117] *(also called B.animalis)* or *Bifidobacterium longum,* to name a few.[118] They should be taken every day, preferably in the evening before you go to bed. When you lie still and are warm and cozy, the bacteria get to work on multiplying and re-establishing the health of your gastro-intestinal system. Speak to your local naturopath or health food store about finding the best probiotic for you, or visit kalebrock.com for helpful links to online suppliers.

Generally speaking, probiotics can be quite safe to take in moderate doses, so take them as suggested on the label of your product. It may be fine to experiment with higher doses for better effect, but ensure this is safe to do so by working with your practitioner.

Make sure you brush your teeth after taking probiotics, as they may affect your enamel. (Capsules are fine.)

Bovine Colostrum

By far one of nature's most complete foods, colostrum is a fundamental tool we can use to assist the healing of our gut lining. You'll recall earlier that we spoke of babies being born with a leaky gut and after receiving nutrients from Mom's colostrum the gut is sealed up. Well, colostrum is actually *very similar (*nutritionally) across all mammalian species—so rather than harvesting colostrum from new mothers around the world (that'd be interesting), we can harness the power of *bovine* colostrum, which comes from cows.

The use of colostrum extends back centuries. Indians would harvest colostrum for medicinal purposes. In Scandinavian countries, the birth of a calf was celebrated, and pudding was made out of the colostrum that was left over after the newborn calf had its share.

> "In addition to containing a high concentration of maternally-derived immunoglobulins, first-milking bovine colostrum is a complex resource of biologically active substances necessary to support the development and repair of cells and tissues; to assure the effective and efficient metabolism of nutrients; and to initiate and support the immune system."[119]
> —A. Fox, Ph.D. and A. Kleinsmith, Ph.D.

Colostrum is such an important part of a cow's (and any mammal for that matter) early hours of life that when calves don't receive it, they often die of an infection. Although we can gather colostrum from cows, the product is *far* from traditional cow's milk, to which many people are sensitive. First of all, the lactose content of colostrum is only 10-15% whereas in milk it is at least 30%. When compared with milk, colostrum contains 10 times more vitamin A, three times more vitamin D, at least 10 times more iron and significantly higher amounts of calcium, phosphorous, and magnesium.[120][121]

Gut protective substances in colostrum, such as IgG, IgM, IgA, and other immune factors, can work within the gut to help fight off infections of pathogenic bacteria and fungi. Lactoferrin and transferrin are particularly interesting nutrients in colostrum; both are mineral-binding carrier proteins which attach to iron, thus starving pathogenic bacteria and yeast. Colostrum has been shown in scientific studies to help control H. pylori, E. coli, and Salmonella infections, along with aiding the healing of Crohn's disease and the gut lining.[122][123][124]

When looking for a colostrum supplement, ensure that it is a high-quality, *therapeutic and pharmaceutical grade* product. Speak to your local naturopath or health food store about finding the best colostrum product for you, or visit kalebrock.com for helpful links to online suppliers.

Dosages will be recommended on your colostrum product.

There is some debate amongst scientists and researchers as to whether the IGF-1 in colostrum* can exacerbate cancer-cell proliferation and tumor growth. Although this is not a settled argument, it is recommended that if you have cancer, you should not ingest colostrum. Speak to your doctor if you still wish to include colostrum in your program.

A special note for athletes—ingesting too much colostrum may result in positive testing for IGF-1.

*https://www.ncbi.nlm.nih.gov/pubmed/18443138

Aloe Vera

As an alternative to colostrum for those who are either very allergic to dairy food or following vegan/vegetarian principles, Aloe vera may be used to reduce inflammation within the GI tract and to assist in healing. Aloe vera can also be used as a prebiotic.[125] The mucilaginous gel in Aloe contains powerful healing properties, however be aware that it does carry a laxative effect on the host (especially the unprepared host). Aloe vera may be particularly helpful in healing inflammatory/acidic conditions of the gut like ulcerative colitis and gastritis.[126]

Take Aloe vera fresh (ensure you have access to edible varieties), or bottled in a high-quality therapeutic food-grade supplement.

Minerals and Trace Elements

Specifically for gut health, minerals and trace elements provide incremental benefits, however I couldn't leave them out of the book. Minerals and trace elements are essential in the optimal functioning of the human body *and although I have not listed them as a gut-essential supplement*, you should consider taking them if you can.

In her book *Colloidal Minerals and Trace Elements*, Dr. Marie-France Muller paints an extraordinarily intricate picture of the body's need for 72 minerals and trace elements per day, pointing out that most people, even those eating a clean, organic diet, are coming up significantly short of this number.

> *"The fact remains that in order to function well our body, just like that of all plants and animals, needs a balanced and sufficient quantity of all this planet's minerals in a form that can be absorbed and assimilated."*
> —*Dr. Marie-France Muller*[127]

The unfortunate reason we are becoming so depleted in this area of nutrition is due principally to the erosion of topsoil and the lack of remineralization processes like flooding, volcanic eruptions, and tidal waves. Our move from growing food on the banks of rivers to dusty plains with very little soil biodiversity has had a large impact on us, the end consumer. We have an abundance of fuel-rich food with a marked lack of nutritional information in it, and according to experts, this is one of the root causes of our current state of health.

> *"No cellular function can be produced correctly if the body isn't receiving all the minerals and trace elements the metabolism needs... It so happens that all degenerative diseases originate, to one degree or another, in a severe mineral depletion of the body."*
>
> —*Dr. Robert LaFave*[128]

Dr. Linus Pauling, the man famous for pioneering information on vitamin C, was focused intently on minerals and their role in health.

> *"You can trace every sickness, every disease, and every ailment to a mineral deficiency."*
>
> —*Dr. Linus Pauling*[129]

And so was Dr. Charles Northern, all the way back in <u>1934</u>:

> *"In the absence of minerals, vitamins have no function. Lacking vitamins, the system can make use of the minerals, but lacking minerals vitamins are useless... Bear in*

mind that minerals are vital to human metabolism and health—and that no plant or animal can appropriate to itself any mineral which is not present in the soil upon which it feeds... The alarming fact is that foods—fruits and vegetables and grains—now being raised on millions of acres of land that no longer contains enough of certain needed minerals, are starving us—no matter how much of them we eat!"

—Dr. Charles Northern[130]

Needless to say, I believe that this is an area of our nutrition that *everybody* should be supplementing. The products you should look for must be a colloidal source of minerals and trace elements and contain at least the 72 we need per day to function optimally. Ideally, they should be sourced from pristine environmental areas. Obtaining these nutrients from a tablet or non-plant source is not the best way to invest your money either, as the bioavailability and usefulness of synthetic minerals is lacking. Remember colloidal (plant-based) minerals and trace elements are 7,000 times smaller than a red blood cell, meaning they have a bioavailability rating of 98%.[131]

"In both the human and the animal body, the bioavailability of nonorganic mineral food supplements is only 8 to 12 percent on average, which falls to 3-5 percent among people who are over the age of 40."[132]

—Dr. Marie-France Muller

A cheap way to obtain these minerals in your diet is through drinking a solution of Himalayan salt in the mornings, however this is not as ideal as obtaining them through colloidal forms due to the bioavailability factor (being much higher in a colloidal state). If you're on a tight budget or cannot access high-quality colloidal mineral supplements, this may be your best option.

Mix one teaspoon of Himalayan salt into a glass of spring water until dissolved. Drink this solution.

My personal issue with this process is it leads to frequent nosebleeds, an indication of an imbalanced (too thin) blood supply, which is the salt's doing. If you are on blood-thinning medication, using this type of salt solution would be dangerous and ill-advised. As such, I choose colloidal minerals and trace elements.

Specifically, minerals and trace elements may assist the cells of your gut lining to begin healing and to function optimally. Bismuth is one trace element that works specifically on the gut lining and has traditionally been used to inhibit the overgrowth of H. pylori. Supplementing minerals and trace elements will also help you stay on top of your cravings as the body becomes nutrified. Often food cravings are actually mineral cravings (or water cravings), and yet up in the brain we hear the message "eat that candy bar now."

Supplementing with recommended dosages (as per the product you buy) twice per day is a good way to start.

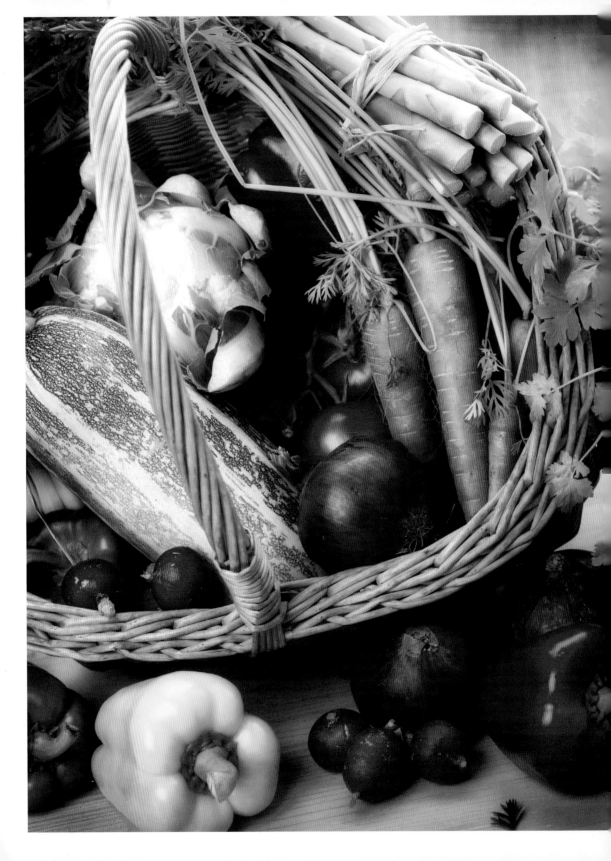

CHAPTER 6

Frequently Asked Questions

Q. *Why not supplement with glutamine?*

There is some evidence that suggests cancer cells can thrive off glutamine, hence my apprehension to recommend it. One of the premises of this protocol is that eating whole foods to create a natural balance of beneficial bacteria in the gut should be used to heal the body.

Q. *Difference between pre- and probiotics?*

Prebiotic refers to the sugar (carbohydrate) molecules which probiotics feed upon—these sugars may also be called insoluble fibers. Probiotics are the living microbes which benefit your body; they're always hungry for good quality prebiotics which come from numerous healthy foods like carrots, onions, beets, greens, and more.

Check out this site for a list of more prebiotic foods: https://draxe.com/prebiotics/

Q. *I'm on the FODMAP diet.*

FODMAP is an acronym for Fermentable Oligosaccharides, Disaccharides, Monosaccharides, and Polyols. These are carbohydrate compounds that are poorly absorbed in some people's digestive systems, meaning they travel through to the large intestine only to feed bacteria (often pathogenic) and produce symptoms of IBS (Irritable Bowel Syndrome).

There are many people who have gone on the FODMAP diet with some success. Although the FODMAP diet is fantastic at reducing or even eliminating the symptoms of IBS like bloating, distension, flatulence, and pain, it fails to address the underlying cause of the issue which is a lack of or inactivity of GLUT-5 transporter proteins that help the small intestine absorb fructose. (It may also be a diet that is *too high* in fructose.) This is significant because GLUT-5 activity is heavily influenced by inflammation within the digestive tract![133]

Probiotics can help in two ways in this situation: 1) they can "eat" the fructose for you and better prepare carbohydrates for the small intestine, and 2) they can work to reduce the level of inflammation within the digestive tract, which may just reactivate the GLUT-5 transporter proteins (more research is needed on this).

During this protocol, it is advised you follow the recommendations of the practitioner who prescribed FODMAP for you, as many of the foods on this protocol are low in FODMAPS anyway. Changing ingredients to replace FODMAPS in recipes will have minimal effect on the recipe's palatability.

Q. I've got constipation on the protocol.
Due to alterations in gut flora and a change in diet, sometimes people do see a die-off reaction whereby constipation may become an issue. To correct this, it is recommended that you include green smoothies in your regime either in addition to meals or as a meal replacement. Also, be sure you focus on chewing food thoroughly and mindfully, adhere to the rules of food combining, drink enough water, exercise, include probiotics, and moderate animal protein intake. You may also need a chiropractic adjustment.

Check that you are covering all these bases, and if symptoms persist, see a doctor or therapist about natural laxatives like Aloe vera.

For an additional detox and constipation intervention, you can try soaking two tablespoons of chia seeds in spring water for 5-10 minutes and then consuming the jelly-like substance.

Q. My symptoms are getting worse on this protocol.
This protocol is not here to treat or cure your illness—it would be illegal and wrong for me to write that. BUT, it is a protocol that has worked very well for numerous people in the past. Sometimes, symptoms do get worse during the time on the GHP; this is known as a Herxheimer reaction, where the body begins to reverse its way along your health journey, dealing with issues it may not have been ready to in the past. Often, symptoms are minor and go away within 1-2 weeks of being on the program, but of course I recommend you see your doctor to help you clarify whether staying on the program is safe.

Keep in mind it is most often the first 2 weeks of a gut-healing journey that are the most challenging. Energy levels often fluctuate, headaches may occur, and cold- and flu- like symptoms may arise. The key is to monitor your health over time to ensure your own safety and know that your body is normally just "getting stuff done" that it wasn't able to before.

Q. I've been diagnosed with SIBO (Small Intestinal Bacterial Overgrowth), and/or I experience constant bloating even on the protocol.
This is where it may be permissible for you to adopt more of a GAPS-style diet while you get control of your condition.

It may be a good idea to reduce the amount of salads and prebiotics in your diet for now, as prebiotics have been shown to be potentially irritating for SIBO and other specific gastrointestinal disorders.[134] By incorporating a more "GAPS"-style approach that focuses on easily digested, healing foods like the broths and soups in this book, you can take the pressure off your GI tract and still remain on this program. Eating these broths and soup-style recipes three times per day for 1-2 weeks should help you overcome your symptoms and kick off your reset program. Green smoothies can be consumed if they do not cause irritation, as they will help add raw, live food into your diet.

Do this until you have regained control of your symptoms, and then slowly reintroduce whole, raw foods back into the diet.

Ensure you take probiotics during this time, and also work with your doctor to see if antibiotic treatment is required. You may require some additional enzyme supplementation while you consume only cooked, soft foods, and it can be a good idea to chew bones to maintain teeth density.

Q. I'm losing weight on the protocol.
Good for you. This is a side-effect of balancing your hormones, microbiome, and fat-burning potential.

Q. I don't want to lose any more weight.
Are you eating enough protein? This is an obvious starting point. The next question should be, are you absorbing/digesting what you're eating? By cutting down on simple carbohydrates in the protocol, we have naturally made you insulin sensitive, meaning you don't need much insulin to shift glucose into your cells every time you eat a carbohydrate. This also means that you will store less fat, as insulin

is also a *storage hormone*. By chewing thoroughly and including pro-biotic supplements, you should be absorbing your protein efficiently. Another important factor is the type of physical training you are doing—you may need to focus less on cardio fitness and more on strength building, anaerobic training.

Q. I've fallen off the program and am struggling to get back on.
That's okay. Take a breath. Often when participants sneak "a little here and there" of the foods not recommended on the protocol, they begin to feel as if they "need" them more and more. This is an emotional response to food and one we want to steer clear of. One of the great benefits of this program (technically speaking; a benefit from being in ketosis and avoiding the blood sugar fluctuations from a standard diet), is that we lose the emotional attachment to food and can go without thinking about it for a long time.

This is actually the sort of state we want to be in during the time on this protocol because it helps us stay on track. I've heard and made all the justifications myself; *trust me.*

"But it's an apple; it's still healthy. Why can't I have that? That's stupid."

Remember, we are attempting to reset your microbiome and gut lining, so for a little while we need to restrict any foods that may potentially have a negative effect on these areas. Yes, an apple, or a little raw treat, or a dark chocolate, may be somewhat healthy for someone with a balanced healthy microbiome, but until that is you, it's best to wait. The body will not die of a sugar deficiency.

Often if you're really struggling to get back on track—just set a new date to start again. Think back to your big WHY, and go from there.

Q. I've got sugar cravings.

This is normal and can be alleviated by following this protocol.

1. Take a drink of water.

Still craving?

2. Have 3-4 almonds and chew thoroughly.

Still craving?

3. Take a pinch of Himalayan salt and let it dissolve on your tongue.

Still hungry?

4. Drink more water.

You may also choose to increase your supplementary minerals and trace elements, as your body may simply be craving these. Ensuring adequate protein intake will moderate any sugar cravings stimulated by blood sugar drops. Also, are you simply bored? Entertain yourself.

Q. I'm vegan.

I can speak from a place of understanding in this regard because I was once a vegan, too. If you're reading this book, then chances are your microbiome and gut are not where they want to be, so I encourage you to ask yourself *is your vegan diet working for you?* If it isn't, then I encourage you to think about including some animal protein in your diet. Including just eggs (or even better, fish and eggs) will help you complete this program and receive the benefits from doing so.

You have to weigh your reasons for being vegan against the benefits of being healthy. Would you be able to serve the world, including its animals, better if you were in a perfect state of health? I daresay the answer is yes. Vegans must also realize that we are part of a wonderful cycle, and as we leave this earth, we are chewed up and devoured by all the world's wonderful microbes, to be incorporated back into the very plants and animals which sustain us now.

Q. I'm hungry all the time.

Are you exercising a lot? If so, it is fine to eat more of the foods allowed on this protocol. This protocol will never recommend calorie restriction—it is recommended that you eat until you are *comfortably full* (leave around 20% of your stomach empty for digestion to occur).

If you are drinking enough water (remember: 33mls per kg of bodyweight, as noted in the Water section in Chapter 4), breathing, supplementing, and staying mentally active, then you shouldn't be consuming more than your body needs. Boredom is an enemy when it comes to snacking excessively so stay active!

Q. I'm not digesting anything—I feel bloated and uncomfortable.

Refer to previous constipation and SIBO/bloating recommendations.

Q. My doctor/dietitian/therapist says I should stop this protocol.

It is impossible for me to write against the recommendations of your doctor or therapist's advice, so I encourage you to work closely with them and to ask them why they think you'd be better off not doing this protocol. Remember this is a *real food* approach to healing, and if you are following the principles, you'll leave no stone unturned when it comes to macronutrients and most micronutrients. I encourage you to ask yourself the question, too—is your coach getting the results that *you want with your own health*, with their patients, or with themselves?

Q. *When can I start having sweet fruit again?*

After the protocol. Use a slow reintroduction schedule and monitor how your digestion feels after each serving. Do not combine fruits when you first reintroduce them because it is necessary that we identify if any particular fruits are causing GI issues. Remember to follow the rules of food combining, eat fruit alone and on an empty stomach, at least until you are certain that you don't have any issues with it. Then, the odd raw dessert and other tasty treat can be consumed on an irregular basis. Don't be surprised when these foods creep up on you and their frequency in your diet skyrockets without you knowing; stay on top of it and be in control.

You're in charge—not your belly.

During the protocol, you can include fruits like tomatoes, cucumbers, lemons, limes, and avocados.

Q. *I'm pregnant.*

Congratulations! Now, you should see your qualified health practitioner to confirm that doing the GHP during pregnancy is safe. As this is a real-food approach to health and wellness, there *should* be no problems with doing so, and certainly those who have participated in the past have benefited greatly during pre-, mid-, and post-pregnancy on the GHP.

Q. *Babies/young children and the GHP—what's the deal?*

I have to tell you to see a qualified health practitioner to ensure the GHP is safe for your child. Again, as this is a real-food approach to wellness, the GHP should work fine for your child, however please use common sense about implementing it. A young child who has just moved on to solid foods is not a good candidate for the GHP, as there may be too much fiber and too much animal protein for him/her to deal with at that time. Healing a young child's gut should be done under the guidance of your integrative GP or naturopath and should have more focus on targeted supplementation (probiotics, colostrum, minerals) as opposed to drastically altering his or her diet. Breastfeeding is extremely important and offers a lot of protection for the developing gut. Until the age of three, a child's microbiome is quite unstable and shifts easily, so any drastic change in diet or supplementation will make a significant impact on your child's health (for the good and bad), so please see your practitioner about implementing the GHP and its principles. Children typically have a high energy and capability for healing, so after a short time, you should see improvements in your child's health.

For children with autism and other behavioral issues, refer to Dr Natasha Campbell-McBride's book: *Gut and Psychology Syndrome*.

If your child is already eating a "standard" diet, then he or she may be a great fit for the GHP as long as you individually tailor portion sizes of food and supplements and take a logical approach.

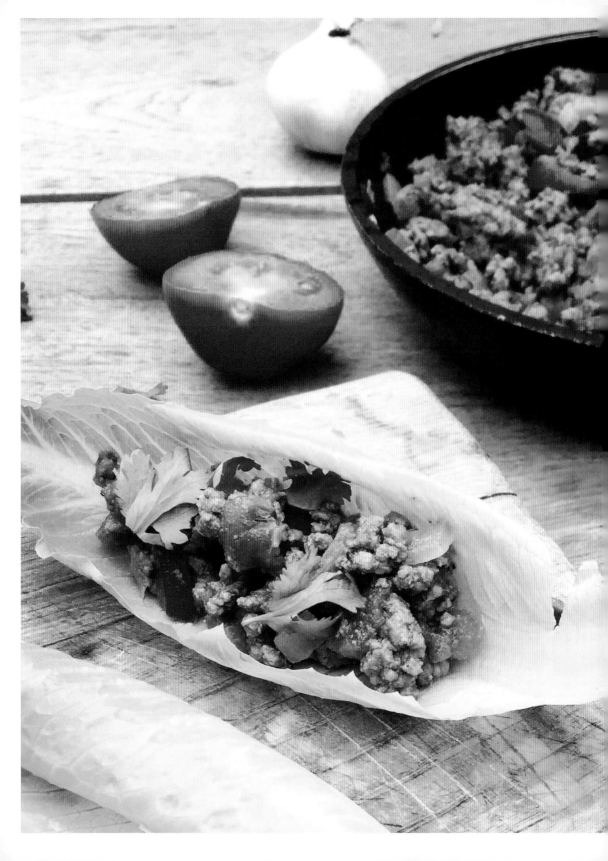

CHAPTER 7

The Recipes

So, you've committed. You've paid for this book, you've (hopefully) created some social accountability by telling your friends, and you're ready to knuckle down and do it.

I recommend that you pick a day on the calendar that you know will work for you in terms of creating new habits. Monday is the common choice for most people because it means they're coming off a weekend of "relaxation." Use your weekend to prepare for the protocol by doing the shopping and making a big salad. If you would like to participate in the transition week before the protocol, then obviously you'll need to factor this into your plans.

I do encourage you to mark on the calendar your 8- to 12-week commitment to this protocol, and I encourage you to share it with your friends to create some accountability for yourself. For social media accountability tools, head to www.kalebrock.com.au/ghp.

Transitioning

The transition week is incredibly important in our protocol because it actually gives you a taste of how you can expect to feel on the protocol (great!), and it also serves to put in place some healthy habits that we'll need for the protocol.

During transition week, there are two basic premises.

You are going to commit to making sure your first meal of the day adheres to the dietary guidelines outlined in this protocol.

Example: normally upon rising, you might consume cereal with milk, but instead you will have two poached eggs with spinach, tomato, and avocado.

You are also going to optimize your water intake during this time.

Example: normally you may go through the day forgetting to drink and at 3:00 p.m. realize you're thirsty. Instead, spread out your water intake throughout the day and consume 33mls per kg* of your bodyweight, plus additional water for exercise. To avoid needing to go to the toilet too much, you can try diluting a small amount of Himalayan salt in your water (not enough to taste it) to increase absorption.

*33mls = 1.11586 ounces / 1kg = 2.20462 lbs.

Again, transition week serves as a nice stepping stone into the actual program; there would be no point overloading you emotionally and physically. There will be participants in the program who actually need this week to allow some light detoxification to take place before they enter the program fully.

In today's day and age, it is important to detoxify slowly and gradually, as overloading the body with too many toxins at one time is extremely dangerous.

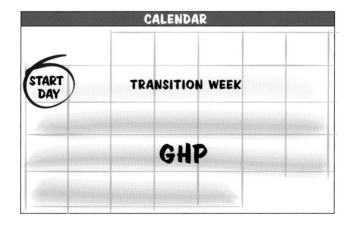

THE GUT HEALING PROTOCOL

You're all set. Enjoy this process. It's really fun feeling great all the time. Let's give you some recipes and sample meal plans to get started.

These recipes have been designed with the Gut Healing Protocol principles in mind. They are perfect guides for you to copy or for you to base your own creations upon. Regardless, enjoy the process of creating healing, nourishing food for yourself and your family.

Breaking from Tradition – An Intuitive Approach to Healing Your Gut

Healing the gut microbiome requires flexibility and using intuition when eating. Many of the traditional breakfast, lunch, and dinner recipes with which we are all familiar are not always appropriate for healing a "leaky gut" or for restoring general gut health.

Following the recipes are two sample menus: the Sample Meal Plan and the Sample Gut Nourishing Meal Plan. The menus are deliberately organized for flexibility. Despite being categorically organized as Breakfast, Snack, Lunch, and Dinner, the recipes suggested in those categories are not necessarily only for a specific meal. For example, the recipes listed for breakfast on the sample menus may include salads or soups as well as more traditional breakfast fare. Also, the sample menus list "leftovers" on several occasions as reminders that you may prepare extra servings of a dish if you would like to cut down on preparation time and you wish to enjoy some leftovers the next day. The sample menus are obviously suggestions, but ultimately the recipes you choose from the Gut Healing Protocol are left up to you.

Recipes are listed in alphabetical order. Bold recipes are included in the Sample Meal Plan and Sample Gut Nourishing Meal Plan found on pages 204 and 215, respectively.

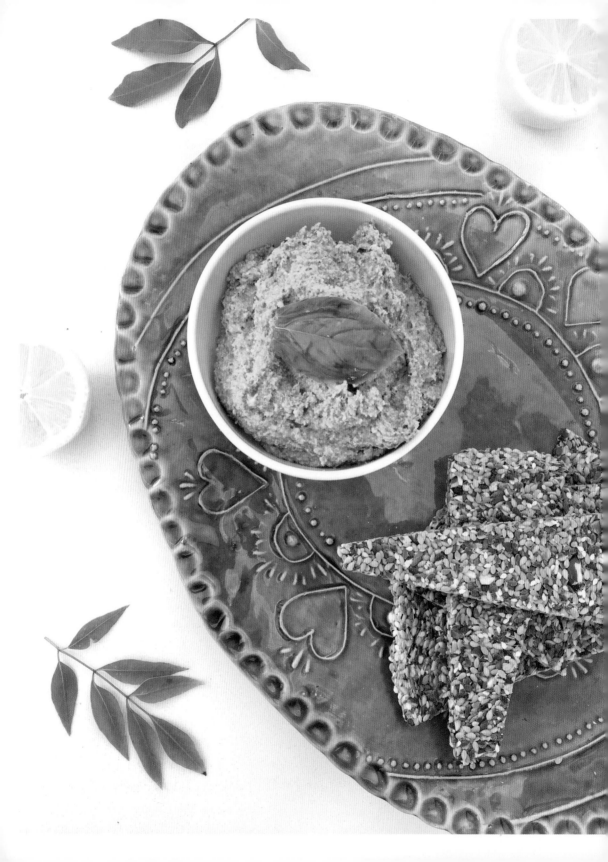

ALMOND BRAZIL PESTO

MAKES 1 LARGE BOWL

INGREDIENTS

1 cup (150 g) Brazil nuts

1 cup (150 g) almonds, soaked for 8 hours then rinsed

1 whole lemon

1/2 bunch parsley

1 bunch basil

1 clove of garlic

1/2 to 1 cup (125 to 250 ml) olive oil

1 teaspoon (5 ml) Himalayan salt

METHOD

Blend all ingredients thoroughly in a food processor until creamy.

Serve on flax crackers or over salad!

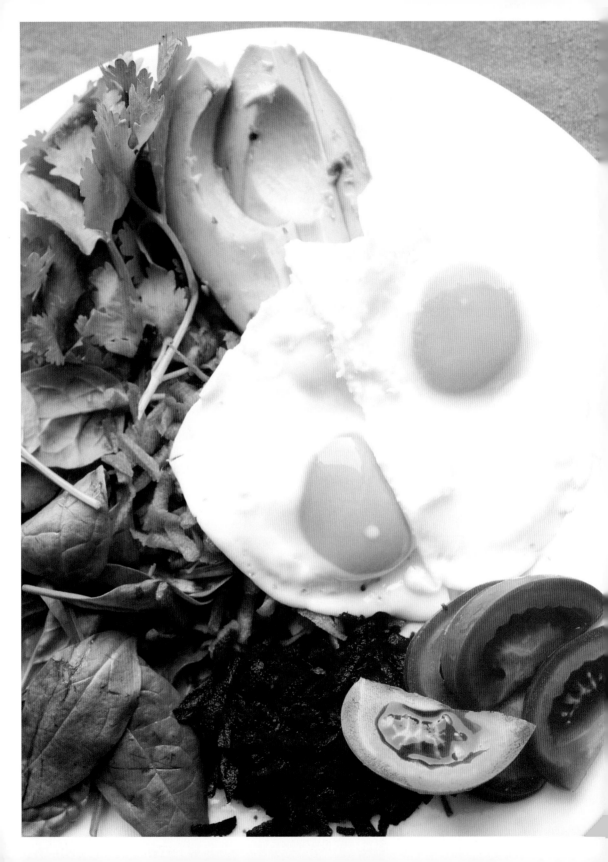

BASIC EGGS

SERVES 1

INGREDIENTS

2 organic eggs

1 teaspoon (5 ml) ghee or coconut oil

1/4 cup (40 g) carrots, shredded

1/4 cup (40 g) beets, shredded

1/2 avocado (optional)

1/2 tomato

1 handful baby spinach

1 small handful of an herb of choice (suggest: cilantro, parsley, or basil)

Pinch of Himalayan salt

Dash of pepper

METHOD

Lightly poach or fry 2 eggs in coconut oil or ghee, keeping the yolk runny.

Shred the carrot and beet, slice the avocado and tomato, and add to the baby spinach on a plate. Once the eggs are cooked, add them to the salad and dress with Himalayan salt, pepper, and herbs.

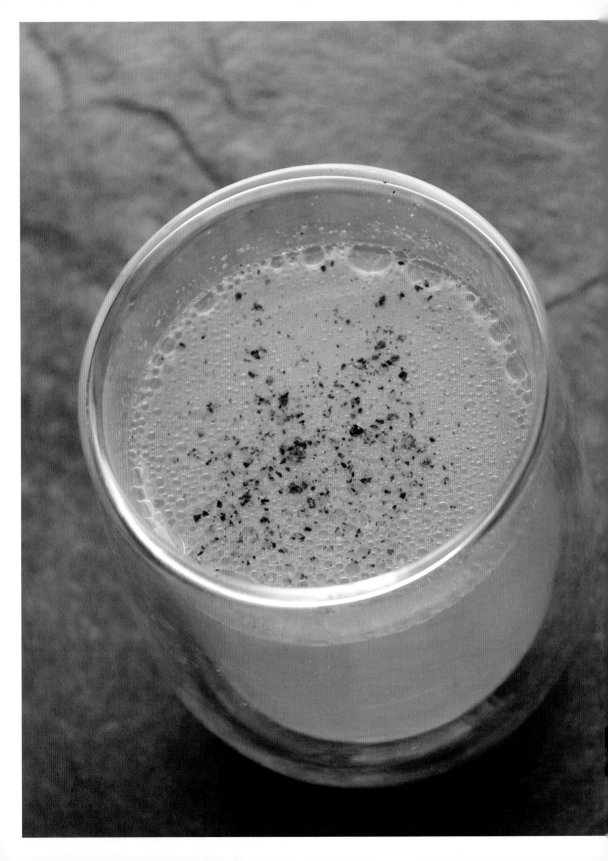

BONE BROTH

MAKES 1.3 GAL (5L)

INGREDIENTS

10 to 15 ounces (300 to 400 g) bones from either lamb, chicken, or beef

1 tablespoon (15 ml) Himalayan salt

2 tablespoons (30 ml) apple cider vinegar

5 quarts (4 to 6 L) spring or filtered water

Optional: carrots, kale, celery, ginger, turmeric, garlic, onion, leek, peppercorns, rosemary, thyme, basil, or parsley.

METHOD

Place all ingredients in a slow-cooker or large saucepan and bring to a low simmer (slightly below boiling point is great). Consider adding carrot tops, kale stalks, celery, ginger, turmeric, garlic, onion, leek, pepper corns, rosemary, thyme, basil, parsley and all manner of flavorsome herbs and spices.

Cover and leave for 18 to 24 hours on a low temperature. To reduce in size and intensify flavor, consider leaving without the lid for 6-8 hours (for ventilation).

Allow the broth to cool before consuming or using as a base for further recipes, as well as before refrigerating.

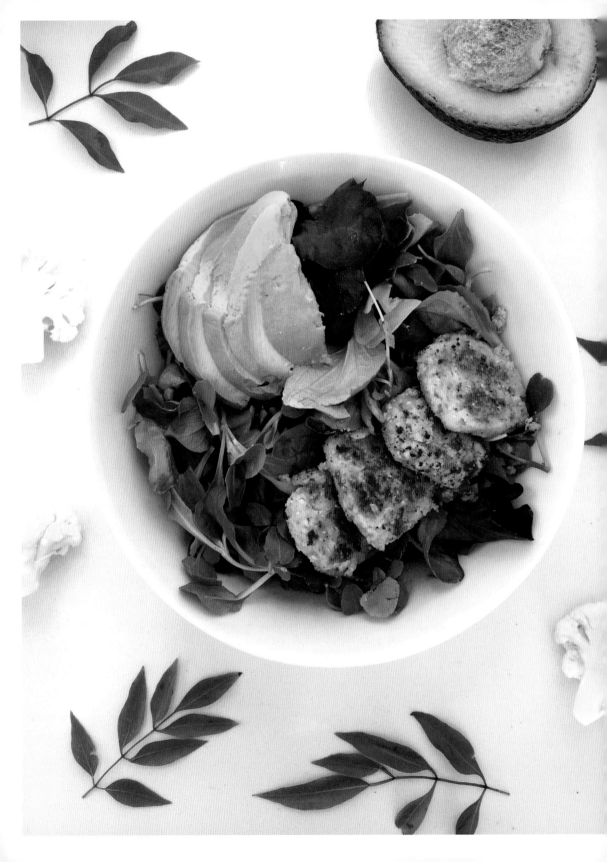

CAULIFRITTERS

MAKES 8 TO 12 FRITTERS

INGREDIENTS

1 medium cauliflower

2 eggs

1 medium red bell pepper

2 cloves garlic

1 medium carrot

2 tablespoons (30 ml) almond meal or flax meal

1/2 teaspoon (2 ml) Himalayan salt

1 tablespoon (15 ml) coconut oil or ghee

METHOD

Blend cauliflower into crumbs in a food processor. Lightly beat the eggs before adding to the processor.

Chop and add the remaining ingredients, except for the coconut oil, to the food processor and blend once more until the desired consistency is achieved.

Using your hands, form the mixture into small patties and then lightly fry, in coconut oil or ghee, until golden. Serve alongside avocado and salad.

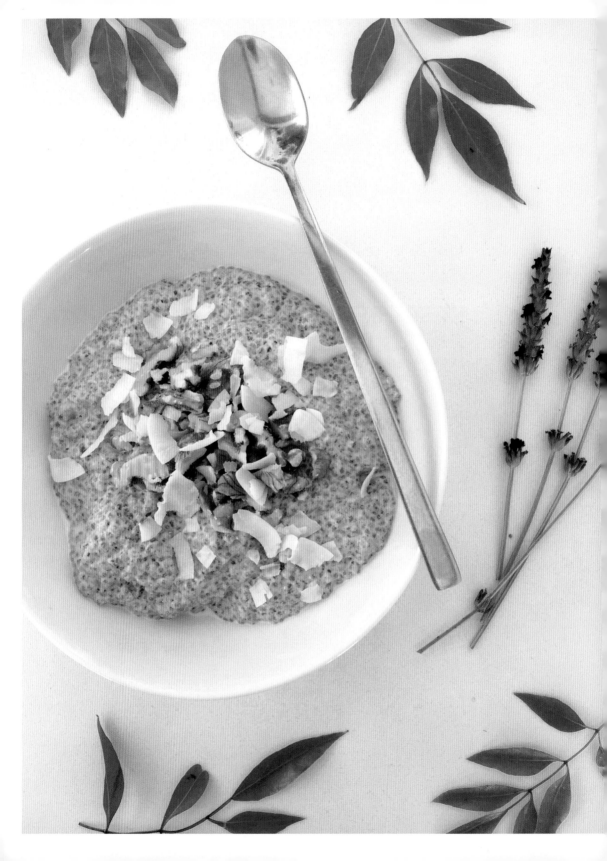

CHIA PUDDING
SERVES 2

INGREDIENTS

1/4 cup (60 ml) chia seeds

1 1/3 cup (325 ml) almond milk (see page 167)

2 teaspoons (10 ml) cinnamon powder

2 handfuls of walnuts

1 handful of coconut flakes

METHOD

Place the chia seeds and 1 cup (250 ml) of almond milk in a small bowl. Mix well to combine, and place in fridge for 1 hour or until the chia seeds have soaked up the milk. You can leave the seeds to soak anywhere from an hour to overnight.

Stir in the cinnamon, walnuts, coconut flakes, and the remaining 1/3 cup (75 ml) of almond (or non-dairy) milk, and serve.

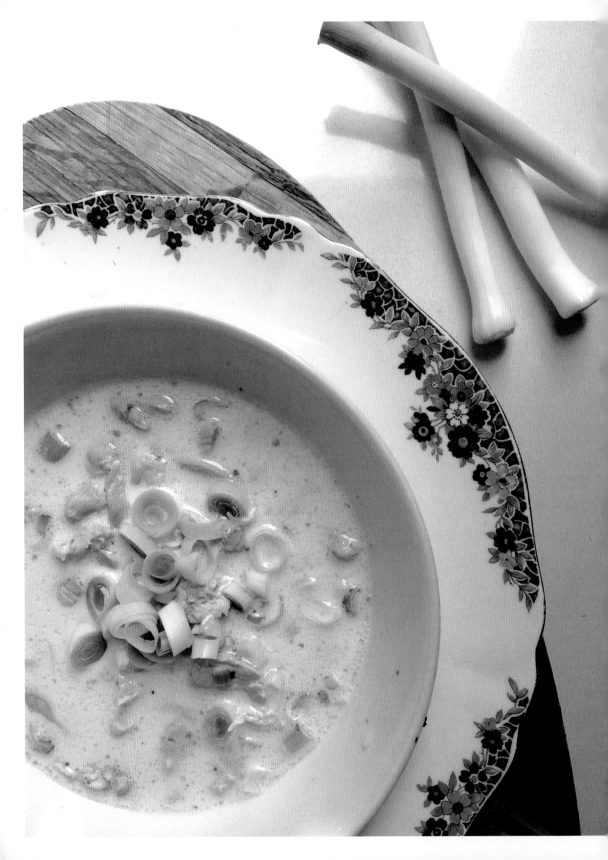

CHICKEN AND LEEK SOUP

SERVES 2 TO 3

INGREDIENTS

1 leek

2 cloves of garlic

14 ounces (400g) cooked chicken pieces (suggest saving the meat from the carcass that is left over from making chicken broth)

1 quart (1 liter) bone broth (preferably chicken)

1/2 cup (125 ml) coconut milk

1 teaspoon Himalayan salt

Dash of black pepper

METHOD

Chop the leek and garlic finely and add along with the remaining ingredients (except the coconut milk and chicken) into a saucepan. Bring to a boil and let simmer for 12 to 15 minutes before adding in the coconut milk and chicken. Allow to sit for a further 3 to 5 minutes while stirring.

Serve warm and keep remainder in the fridge.

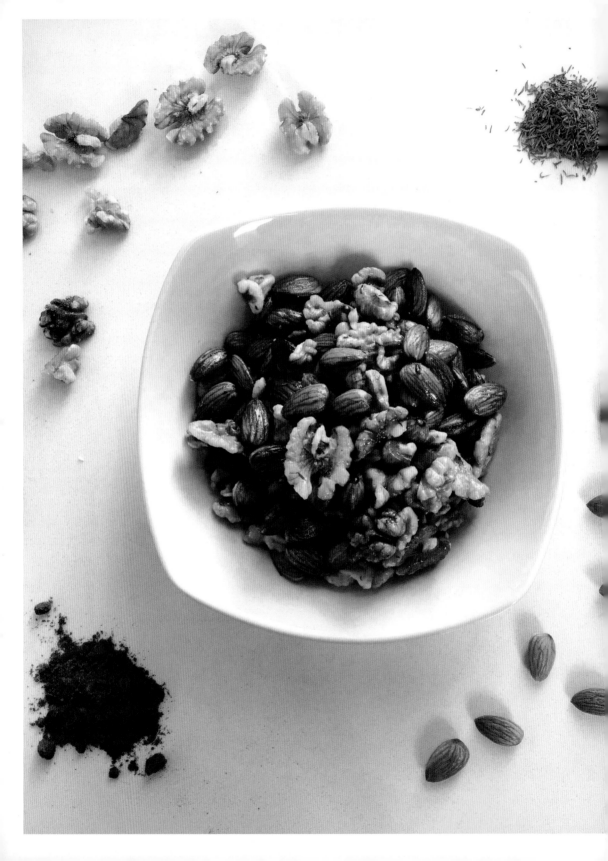

CHILI NUT MIX

INGREDIENTS

1 teaspoon (5 ml) cayenne pepper

1 teaspoon (5 ml) dried thyme

1 teaspoon (5 ml) seaweed flakes of choice (dulse or nori, both are fantastic)

1 tablespoon (15 ml) lime juice

1 teaspoon (5 ml) Himalayan salt

2 tablespoons (30 ml) coconut oil or ghee

3 cups (450 g) walnut/almond mix

METHOD

In a bowl combine the spices, seaweed flakes, and lime juice.

Once thoroughly combined, add nuts to the mix and coat them well before placing them in a dehydrator for 24 hours at 108 degrees F (42 degrees C) or in an oven at 300 degrees F (150 degrees C) for 20 minutes.

You may wish to shake and turn the nuts periodically while dehydrating. Store in an airtight container at room temperature in winter or the fridge in summer.

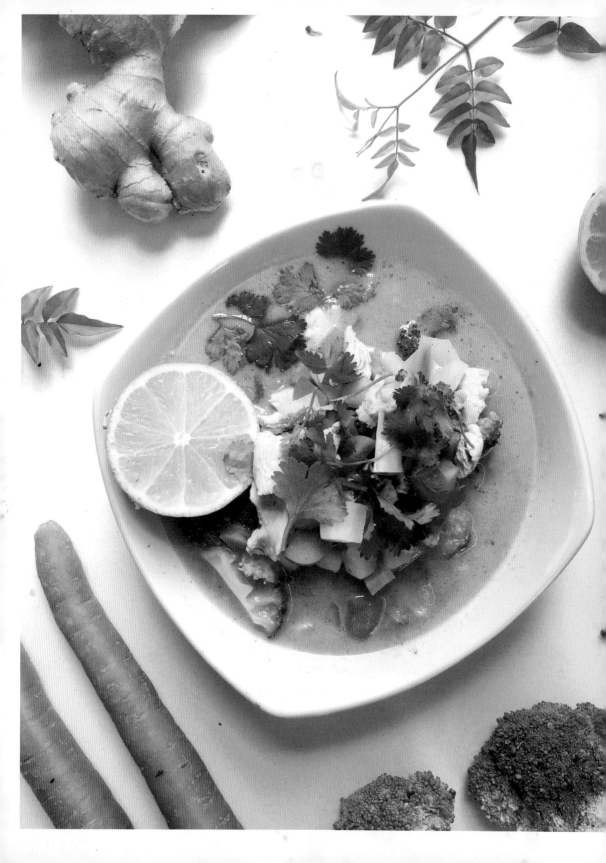

COCONUT LIME CHICKEN SOUP

SERVES 2 TO 3

INGREDIENTS

1/2 cup (125 ml) lime juice

2 carrots

1 medium sweet potato

1 medium head of broccoli

2-inch (5 cm) piece of fresh ginger

1/4 teaspoon (2 ml) cayenne pepper

1/4 teaspoon (2 ml) cinnamon

1 teaspoon (5 ml) Himalayan salt

14 ounces (400 g) cooked chicken

1 can coconut milk

25 fluid ounces (750 ml) bone broth of choice

1 handful of fresh cilantro

METHOD

Chop vegetables as desired. Ginger should be sliced in fine slivers that can be removed before serving, if you wish.

Combine all the ingredients in a saucepan, bring to a boil, and then let simmer for 15 to 20 minutes before serving with fresh cilantro leaves.

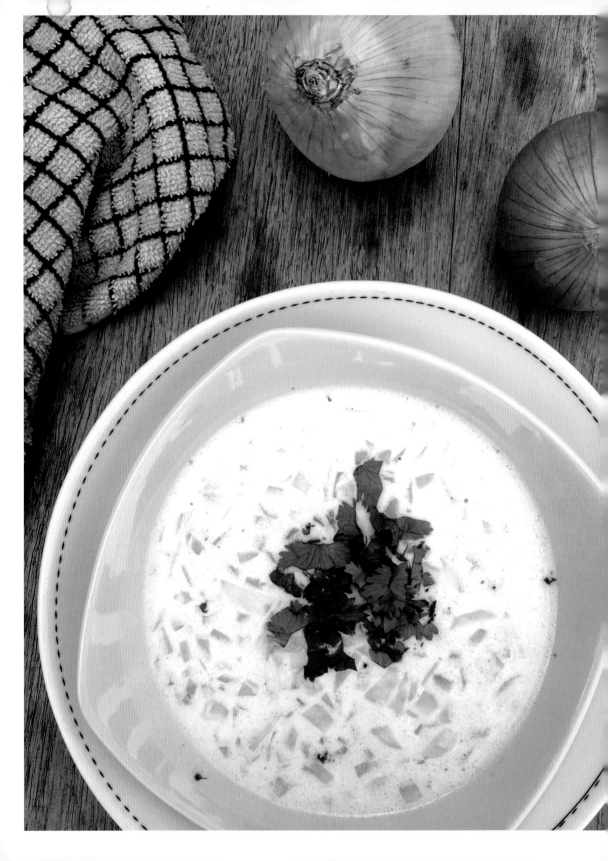

CREAMY ONION SOUP

SERVES 2

INGREDIENTS

4 onions

1 teaspoon (5 ml) apple cider vinegar
(allowed in the Gut Healing Protocol when cooked)

1 quart (1 liter) of bone broth of choice

4 tablespoons (60 ml) of olive oil or ghee

1/2 cup (125 ml) coconut milk

1 teaspoon (5 ml) Himalayan salt

Dash of black pepper

METHOD

Chop the onions finely and add, along with all other ingredients
except coconut milk, to a saucepan. Bring to a boil and let simmer
for 20 to 25 minutes before adding in coconut milk and stirring.

Serve warm and keep remainder in the fridge.

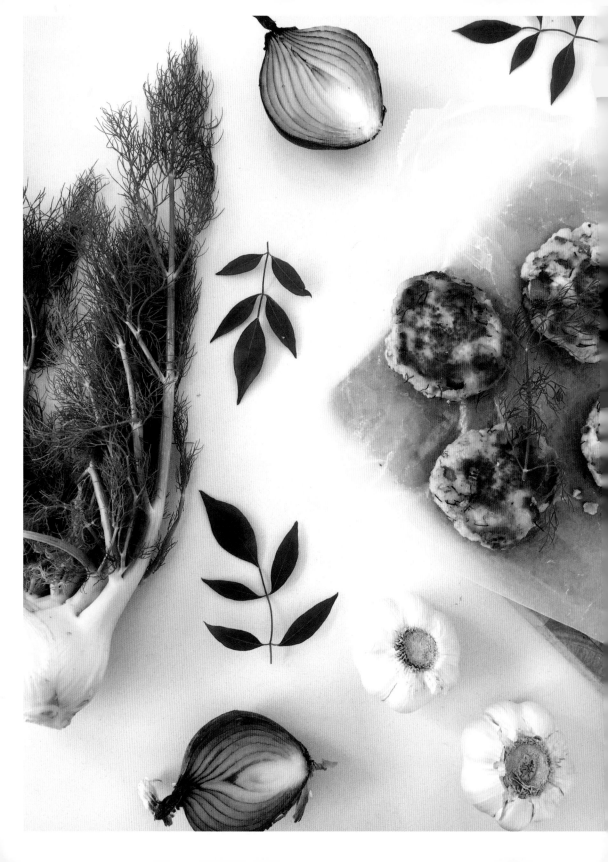

FENNEL FISH FRITTERS

MAKES 8 TO 12 FRITTERS

INGREDIENTS

1 fennel bulb

2 eggs lightly beaten

1 tablespoon (15 ml) coconut flour

1/2 red onion

2 tablespoons (30 ml) fresh dill

1/2 teaspoon (2 ml) turmeric powder

1/2 teaspoon (2 ml) ground black pepper

1 tablespoon (15 ml) coconut oil

1 teaspoon (5 ml) Himalayan salt

5 ounces (150 grams) fresh fish

METHOD

Lightly beat the eggs.

Combine the remaining ingredients in a food processor, including the fish, creating as chunky a mixture as you like. Mix well with the eggs.

Using your hands, create small burger patties out of the mixture and fry on low heat until cooked through on both sides.

Serve with salad.

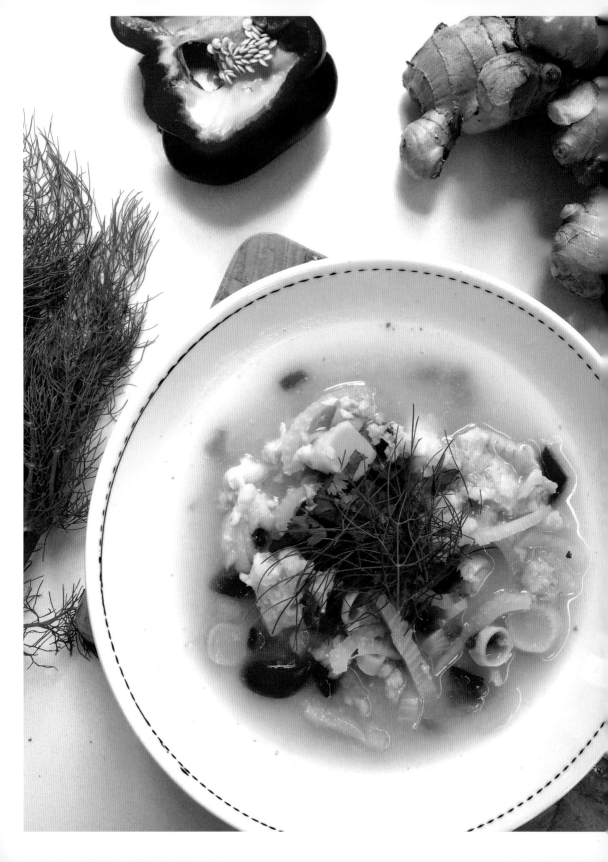

FISH SOUP

SERVES 2-3

INGREDIENTS

14 ounces (400g) snapper, whiting, or your favorite fish

2-inch (5 cm) piece of ginger

1 tablespoon (15 ml) lemongrass

1 red pepper

1/2 small fennel bulb

25 fluid ounces (750ml) bone broth (fish bones work well)

1 teaspoon (5 ml) Himalayan salt

Dash of black pepper

Parsley for garnish

METHOD

Chop fish into cubes. Chop ginger finely into slivers.

Chop vegetables as desired and combine all in a saucepan with bone broth. Bring to a boil and let simmer for 5 minutes.

Add fish cubes to the broth and allow it to simmer for 10 to 15 minutes before serving with fresh parsley.

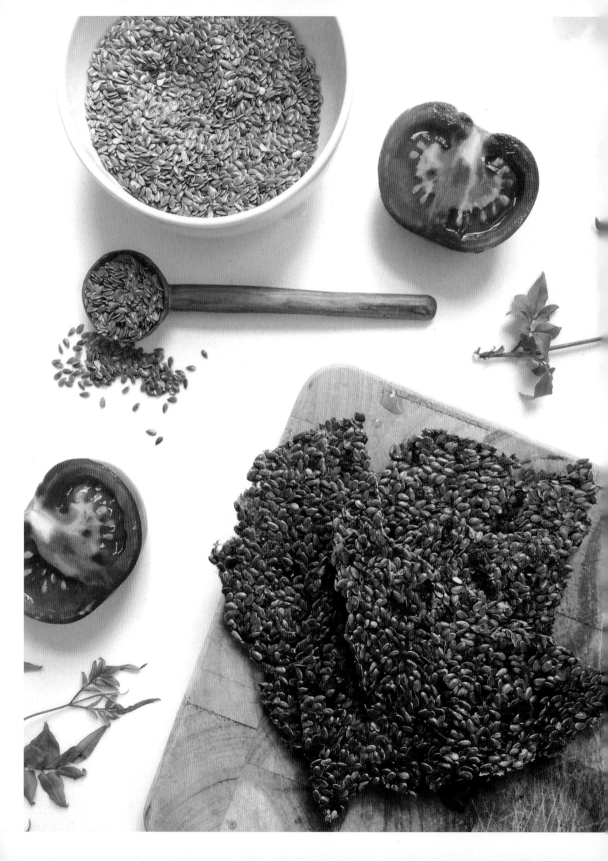

FLAX CRACKERS

MAKES 7 DEHYDRATOR TRAYS

INGREDIENTS

If using an oven, recipe can be halved to allow for space.

17 ounces (500 g) flax or linseeds soaked in water for 20 to 30 minutes

2 cloves of garlic

4 tomatoes

2 red bell peppers

1 handful of arugula

1 tablespoon (15 ml) Himalayan salt

Italian herbs and spices, to taste

METHOD

To make the crackers, blend all ingredients, including the soaked flax seeds, in a blender into a very thick smoothie. You might want to blend the vegetables and herbs first before adding the seeds.

Using a dehydrator, spread the cracker mix onto the sheets about 3/4 inch (1/2 cm) thick and let dry at 108 degrees F (42° Celsius) for 24 hours, flipping them at 12 hours.

If using an oven, bake at 150 degrees F (60 to 70° Celsius) for 12 hours, flipping at 6 hours. Be careful not to burn the crackers.

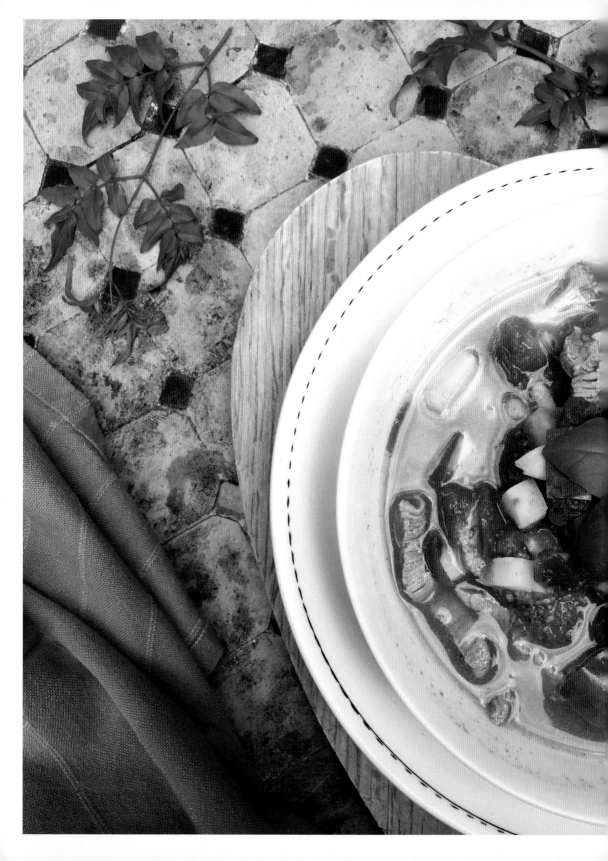

FODMAP-FRIENDLY RED BEEF SOUP
SERVES 2 TO 3

INGREDIENTS

1 medium head of broccoli

1/2 medium sweet potato

2-inch (5 cm) piece of fresh turmeric

1 teaspoon (5 ml) paprika

1 teaspoon (5 ml) cayenne pepper

1 teaspoon (5 ml) Himalayan salt

1 quart (1 liter) bone broth of choice

3 tomatoes

14 ounces (400 g) beef strips (as for stir fry)

1 handful fresh basil

METHOD

Chop and combine vegetables (except tomatoes), herbs, and spices into a saucepan with the bone broth and bring to a light boil.

Simmer for 10 minutes, before adding tomatoes and finally the beef strips. Simmer for another 5 minutes before serving with fresh basil leaves.

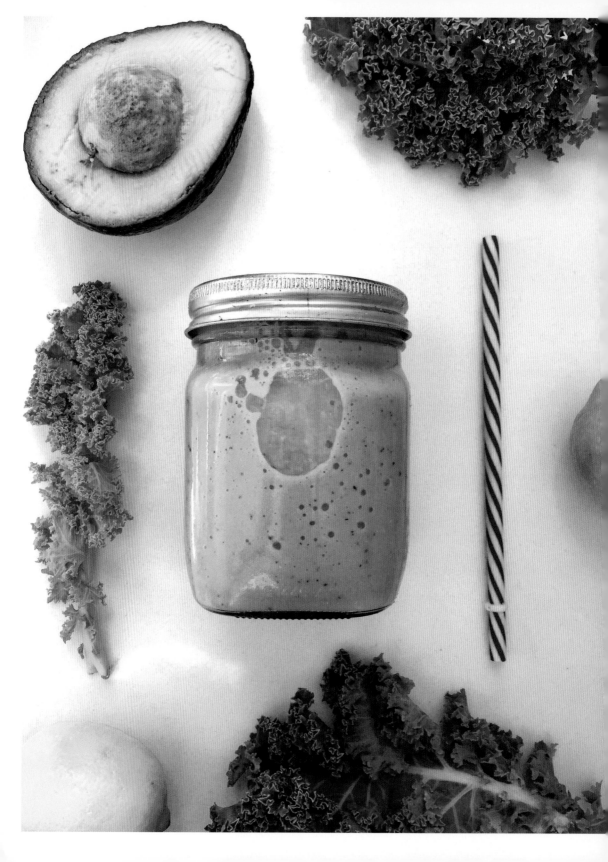

GREEN SMOOTHIE

SERVES 1

INGREDIENTS

2 handfuls of greens (suggest: cilantro, parsley, spinach, kale, basil, or collards)

1 lemon or lime (with some peel)

1 small avocado or 1/4 cup (60 ml) olive oil

2 to 3 cups (500 to 750 ml) of water

METHOD

Place all ingredients into a blender and blend until smooth.

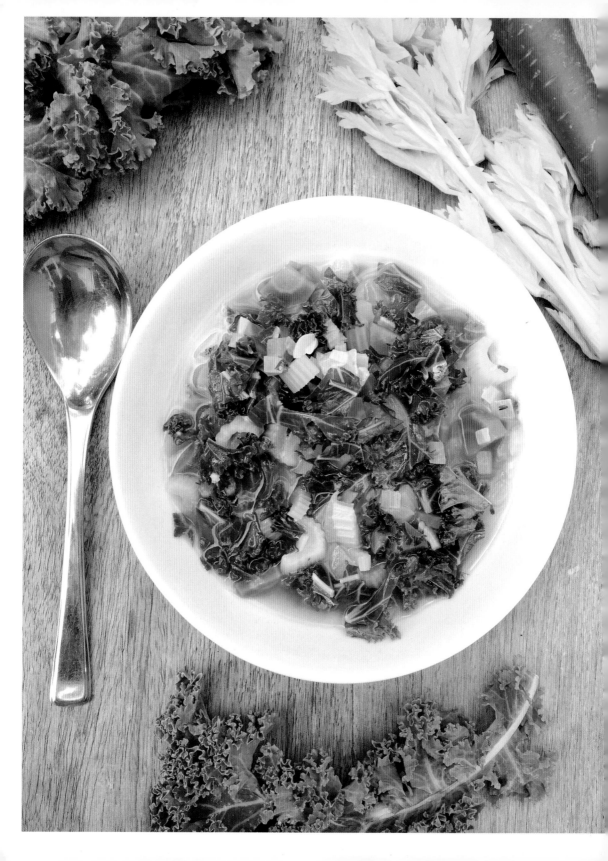

HEALING KALE SOUP

SERVES 2

INGREDIENTS

1 quart (1 liter) of bone broth of choice

1 onion

3 cloves of garlic

1 tablespoon (30 ml) of coconut oil or ghee (optional)

1 carrot

8 kale leaves (stems removed)

3 stalks of celery

2 teaspoons (10 ml) thyme, fresh or dried

1 teaspoon (5 ml) Himalayan salt

Dash of pepper

METHOD

Chop the vegetables to the size you desire.

Place all the chopped ingredients along with the herbs and salt into a saucepan with the bone broth and simmer lightly for 15 to 20 minutes. (Optional: momentarily sauté the garlic and onion in ghee or coconut oil before placing in saucepan—to take the edge off their flavor.)

Serve warm.

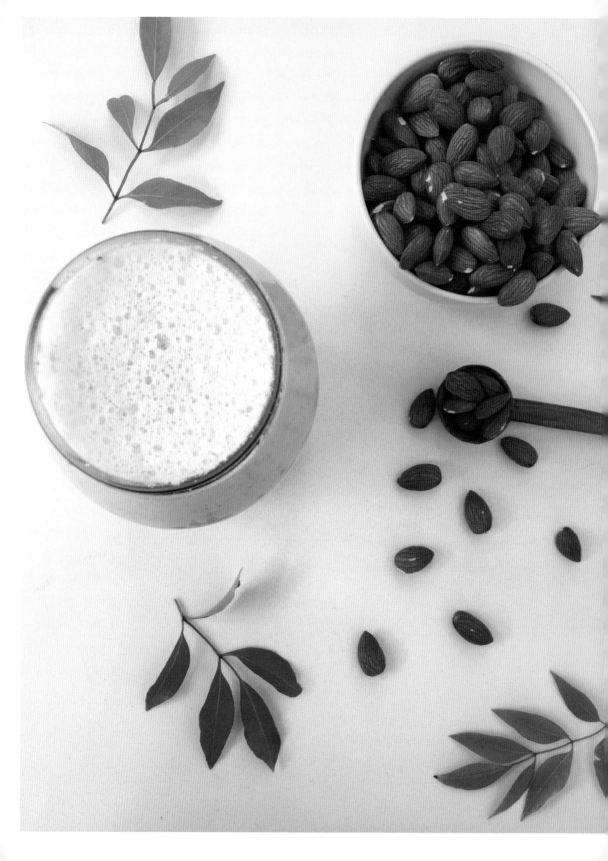

HOMEMADE ALMOND MILK

MAKES 1 QUART (1 LITER)

INGREDIENTS

1 cup (150 g) raw almonds

4 cups (1 liter) water

1⁄2 teaspoon (2 ml) cinnamon

1⁄2 teaspoon (2 ml) vanilla extract/powder

A few drops of liquid stevia (optional)

METHOD

Blend all together in a high-powered blender. To ensure smoothness start off with a little water and slowly add more. You can also filter through a muslin cloth.

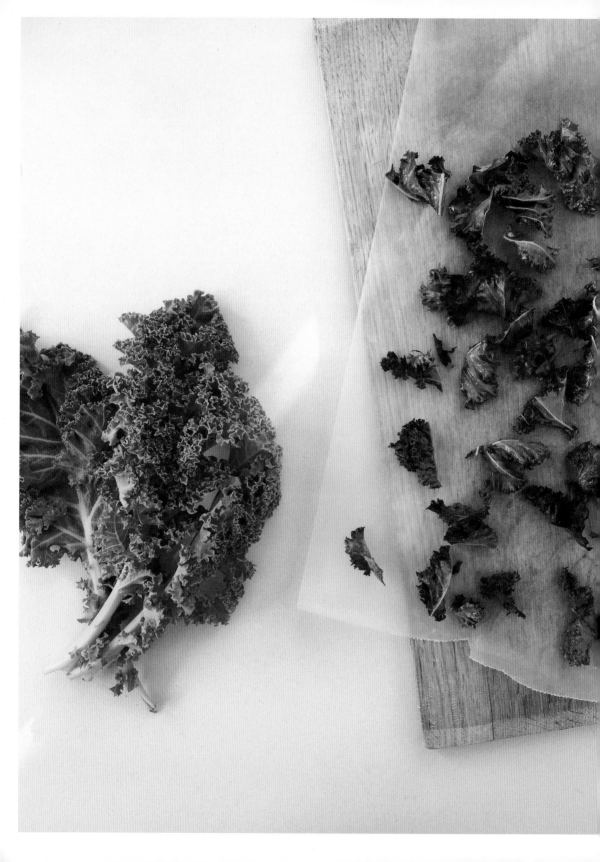

KALE CHIPS

MAKES 1 SMALL BOWL

INGREDIENTS

Handful of kale

Drizzle of olive oil

Himalayan or sea salt to sprinkle

METHOD

Preheat the oven to 350 degrees F (180 degrees C).

Using a knife, separate the leaves from the stalk of the kale. Then cut those leaves into bite-size pieces. Place in a bowl and drizzle with enough olive oil so that it can be rubbed into all the leaves. Add some salt and massage the leaves with your hands until all of them are well coated in oil.

Place on a baking tray lined with parchment paper. Make sure all the leaves are evenly layered out so that none are touching. Leave them in the oven for about 8 minutes (start checking at about 7 minutes). You want them to be crispy but to still maintain their vibrant green.

Alternatively, you can dehydrate them in a dehydrator for 24 hours at 107 degrees F (42 degrees C).

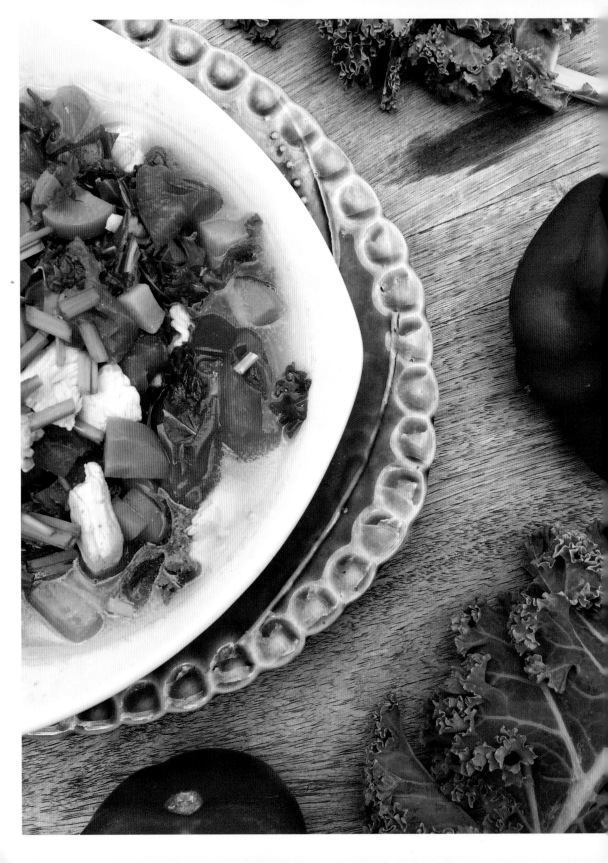

KALE, TOMATO,
AND CHICKEN SOUP
SERVES 2 TO 3

INGREDIENTS

3 carrots

1 red bell pepper

1 teaspoon (5 ml) Himalayan salt

1 quart (1 liter) of bone broth of choice

3 tomatoes

10 kale leaves (stems removed)

1 handful fresh chives

14 ounces (400 g) cooked chicken

Dried basil to taste

Dash of black pepper

METHOD

Chop the vegetables to the size desired and then add the chopped carrots, red bell pepper, and salt along with the bone broth into a saucepan.

Bring the broth and vegetables to a boil and then allow it to simmer.

Add in the tomatoes, kale, chives, and cooked chicken and continue to simmer for 15 more minutes before serving. Dress with dried basil to taste.

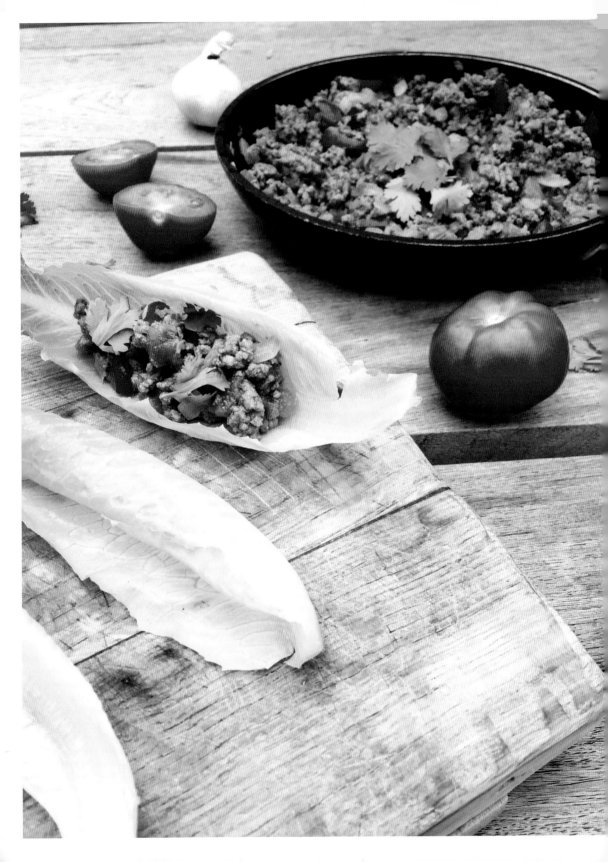

LETTUCE TACOS

SERVES 2

INGREDIENTS

12 ounces (350 g) ground beef

1 onion

1 red pepper

2 cloves garlic

1 tablespoon (15 ml) cumin powder

1 tablespoon (15 ml) oregano

1 tablespoon (15 ml) paprika

1/2 teaspoon (2 ml) cayenne pepper

1 teaspoon (5 ml) Himalayan salt

1 teaspoon (5 ml) ground black pepper

1 tablespoon (15 ml) coconut oil or ghee

3 tomatoes

4 large Romaine lettuce leaves

1/2 bunch cilantro

METHOD

Blend the following ingredients in a food processor until well mixed: onion, bell pepper, ground beef, garlic, cumin, oregano, paprika, cayenne pepper, salt, and black pepper.

Melt one tablespoon of ghee or coconut oil in a covered pan (used for a steaming effect), and lightly cook the vegetable and ground beef mixture for 5 to 7 minutes.

Add the tomatoes to the pan and cook for a further 2 to 3 minutes, ensuring the ground beef is thoroughly cooked.

Drain any water that may have condensed from the mixture. Spoon the taco mixture into your lettuce leaves (instead of tortillas)! Dress with fresh cilantro leaves and enjoy!

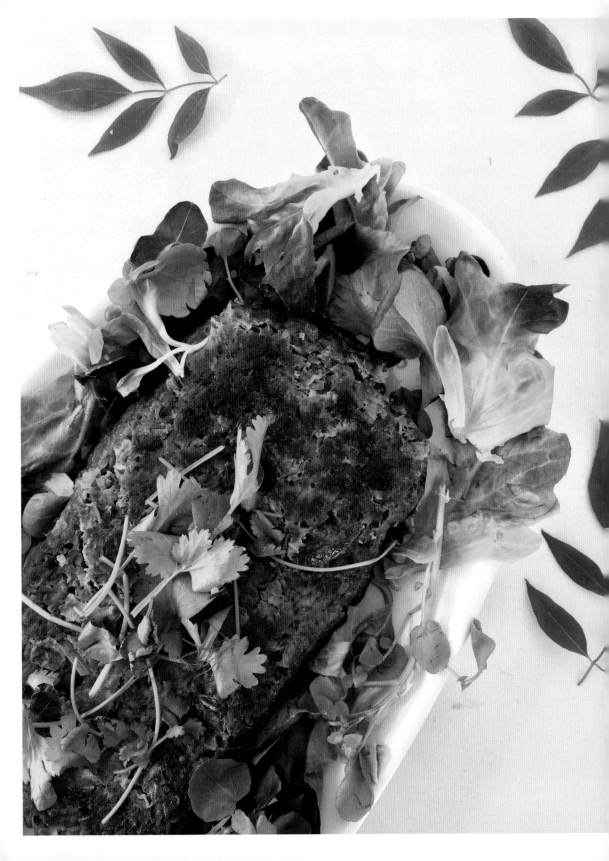

MEATLOAF

MAKES 1 LOAF

INGREDIENTS

10 ounces (300 g) minced grass-fed beef

1 egg, lightly beaten

1 carrot

5 kale leaves, finely chopped

2 garlic cloves

1 big handful of finely chopped basil

1-1/2 teaspoons (7 ml) Himalayan salt

2 teaspoons (10 ml) dried or fresh thyme

METHOD

Preheat oven to 350 degrees F (180ºC).

Blend all ingredients together or mash with hands and place into a loaf pan. Bake in the oven for 60 to 70 minutes until cooked through.

Remove from the oven and allow to sit and cool for 10 to 15 minutes before turning and serving.

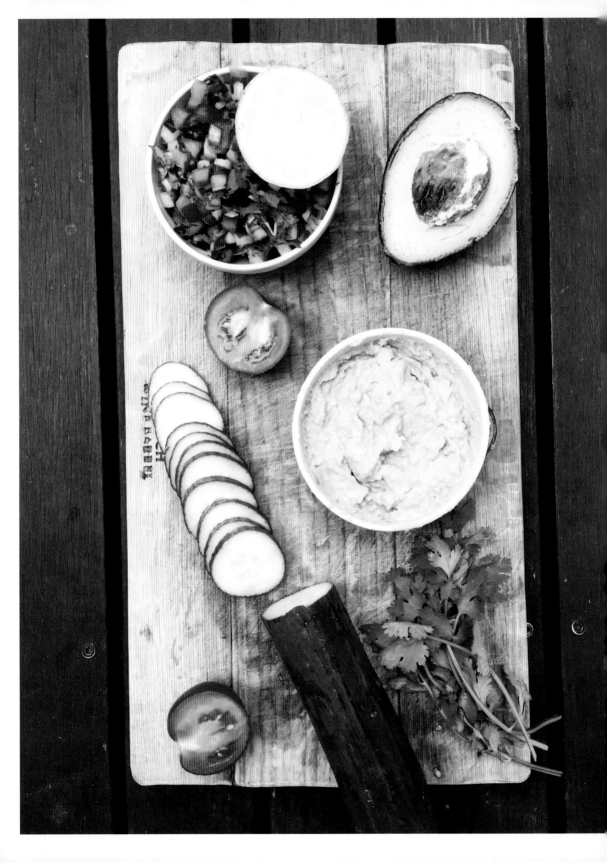

MEXICAN SALSA AND
GUAC WITH CUCUMBER CHIPS

SERVES 2 TO 3

INGREDIENTS

SALSA

6 tomatoes

2 red onions

1 bunch finely chopped cilantro

2 lemons or limes, juiced

1 teaspoon (5 ml) Himalayan salt

1/4 teaspoon (1 ml) black pepper

2 cucumbers, sliced thickly
(for dipping)

1 small jalapeño (optional)

1 teaspoon (5 ml) dulse or kelp
flakes (optional)

GUACAMOLE

2 large avocados

1 lemon, juiced

1 clove garlic crushed

1/2 teaspoon (2 ml) Himalayan salt

METHOD

Finely dice your tomatoes and place them in a bowl. Add your finely chopped onion, cilantro, jalapeño, lemon/lime juice, seaweed flakes, salt, and pepper and toss in a bowl. Let sit for 15 to 20 minutes before serving.

With a fork, blend together the guacamole ingredients until creamy and smooth. A food processor may be used.

Thickly slice the cucumbers for dipping into your salsa and guacamole! Flax crackers may also be used.

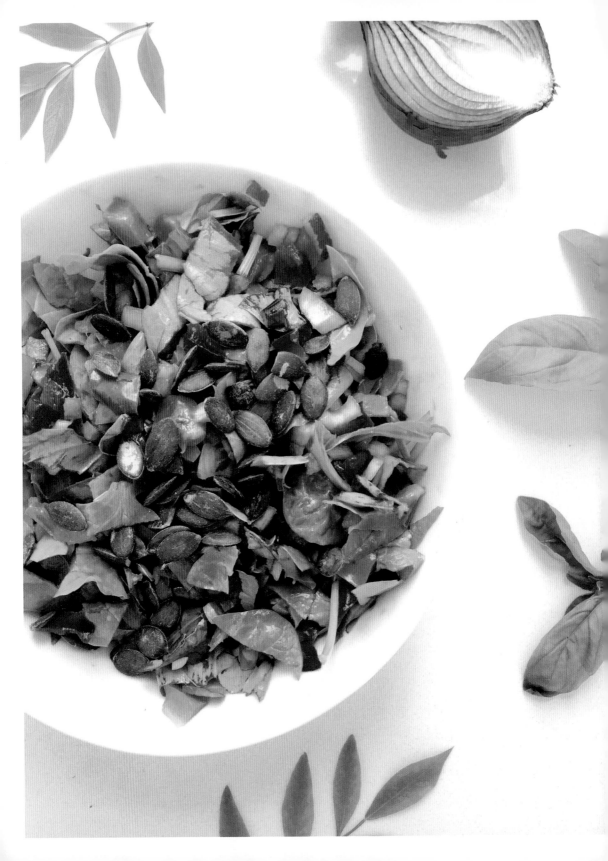

MIXED PEPPER AND BASIL SALAD

SERVES 2

INGREDIENTS

2 red bell peppers

Olive oil

Dash of salt and pepper

1/2 red onion

2 handfuls of fresh baby spinach

2 tablespoons of shredded fresh basil leaves

1 tablespoon of pumpkin seeds

METHOD

Preheat the oven to 350 degrees F (180 degrees C).

Prepare the red bell peppers by slicing off the ends and cutting them in half and removing all the seeds. Place the bell peppers in a baking dish, drizzle with olive oil, and add salt and pepper. Leave the red bell pepper to roast in the oven for about 20 minutes until very soft. Once the red bell pepper is done, allow it to cool and then finely dice and place in a bowl.

Finely dice the red onion and add to the bowl with the diced bell pepper, English spinach, shredded basil, and pumpkin seeds.

Toss the ingredients and serve.

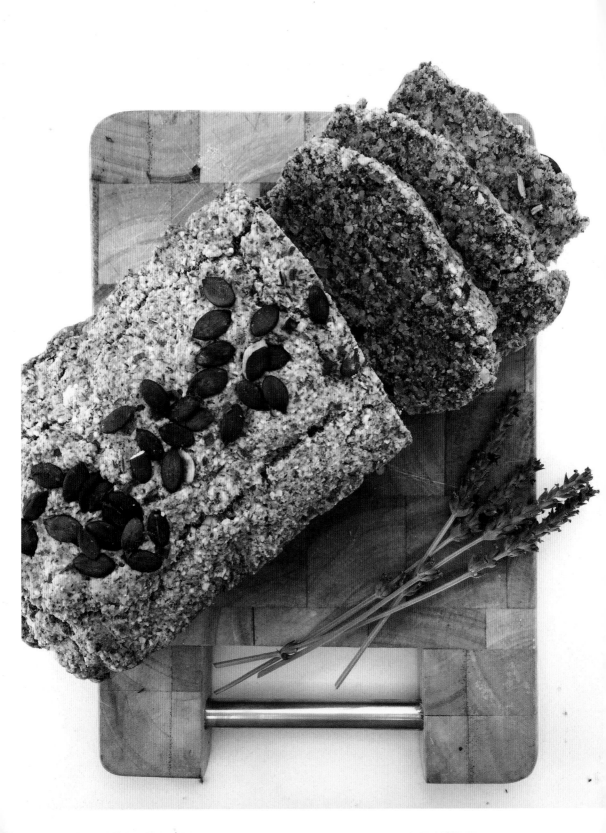

PALEO BREAD

MAKES 1 MEDIUM-LARGE LOAF

INGREDIENTS

1/4 cup (60 ml) coconut oil

5 cups (750 g) soaked almonds
or 4 cups (480 g) almond flour

6 eggs

1 teaspoon (5 ml) lemon juice

1/4 cup (60 ml) ground flax meal

1 teaspoon (5 ml) aluminum-free
baking soda

1/2 teaspoon (2 ml) Himalayan salt

2 teaspoons (10 ml) Italian herbs

2 teaspoons (10 ml) pumpkin seeds

METHOD

Preheat oven to 350 degrees F (175 degrees C).

Line a medium-sized bread pan with parchment paper, and wipe some coconut oil on the paper.

Rinse the soaked almonds under fresh water and drain. Then, in a food processor, blend the almonds until a flour-like consistency is achieved.

Add the liquid ingredients to the food processor—the eggs and lemon juice first—and continue blending, followed by most of the dry ingredients: the flax meal, baking soda, and salt. Save the Italian herbs and pumpkin seeds.

Transfer the mixture into the parchment-lined and lightly oiled bread pan. Dress with Italian herbs and pumpkin seeds, pressing those slightly into the mix, and bake for 35 to 40 minutes.

Remove from the oven and allow to cool for 10 minutes before removing from the pan. This bread keeps in the fridge for 7 to 10 days or in the freezer for 30 days.

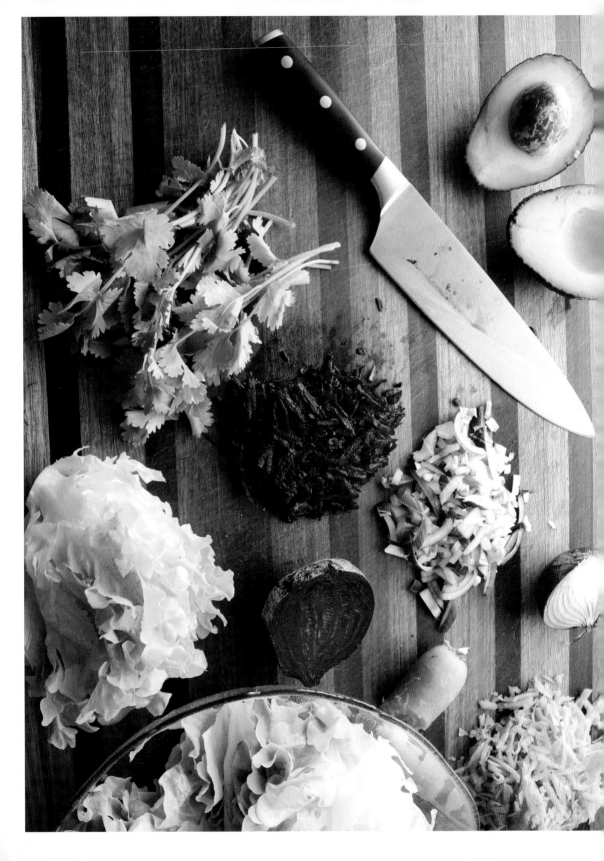

RAINBOW SALAD

SERVES 2

INGREDIENTS

1 carrot

1 beet

1 red onion

1 avocado

1 handful of an herb of choice (suggest: cilantro, parsley or basil)

3 to 4 big handfuls of greens of choice (suggest: lettuce, baby spinach, collards, kale)

1 lemon, juiced

3 to 4 tablespoons (45 to 60 ml) olive oil

Pinch of salt

Dash of pepper to taste

METHOD

Shred the carrot and beet, dice the onion, cube an avocado and chop the herb of choice. Mix all the ingredients in a large salad bowl with the greens of your choice.

For the dressing, squeeze the juice of a whole lemon, then drizzle the olive oil, and add salt and pepper to taste. (If you will be storing some of the salad in the fridge for leftovers, only dress the salad you are consuming to avoid the greens becoming soggy.)

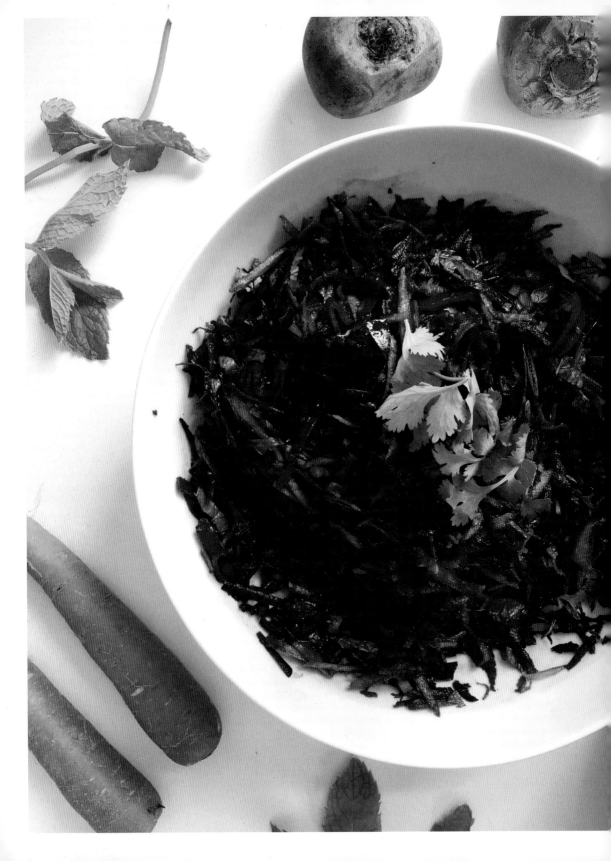

RED PREBIOTIC SALAD

SERVES 2

INGREDIENTS

Purple cabbage (one quarter, chopped)

4 carrots

2 Spanish onions

2 beets

1/2 bunch cilantro

1 handful fresh mint

1/2 cup (75 ml) olive oil

3 whole lemons (peeled)

1-inch (3 cm) piece fresh ginger

1 clove garlic (optional)

1 teaspoon (5 ml) Himalayan salt

1 teaspoon (5 ml) ground black pepper

METHOD

In a food processor, shred cabbage, carrots, onions, beets, cilantro, and mint until you achieve a nice salad consistency. Transfer to a bowl.

DRESSING

In a blender, blend the half cup of olive oil, lemons, ginger, garlic, salt, and pepper into a smooth dressing. (You might need to add extra olive oil depending on the size of your lemons.) Drizzle this over your salad and let sit for 20 to 30 minutes before serving.

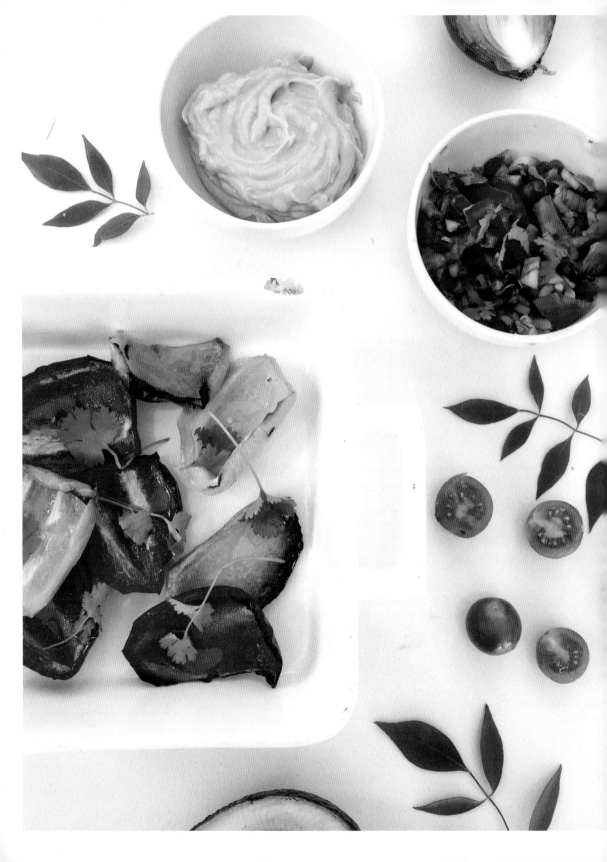

ROASTED BELL PEPPER, AVOCADO CREAM, AND CILANTRO SALSA

SERVES 2

INGREDIENTS

1 medium red bell pepper

2 medium tomatoes

1/2 red onion

1 ripe avocado

1/2 teaspoon (2 ml) ground mustard seeds

1 lemon, juiced

1 handful of fresh cilantro

Drizzle of olive oil

Himalayan salt

Black pepper

METHOD

Preheat the oven to 350 degrees F (180 degrees C). Slice the red bell pepper into discs of about 3/4 of an inch (2 cm) thickness (you want it to be quite thick so that the portions are substantial), then place them in a baking dish, drizzle with olive oil, and sprinkle with some salt. Leave the red bell pepper to roast in the oven for about 20 minutes until very soft. While that is cooking, make the salsa.

FOR THE SALSA

Dice the tomatoes and red onion then combine them in a small bowl with cilantro leaves and half the lemon juice.

FOR THE AVOCADO CREAM

Blend the avocado, black pepper, and the other half of the lemon juice with the mustard seeds until it forms a smooth, creamy consistency. Serve over the roasted red bell peppers and top with the salsa.

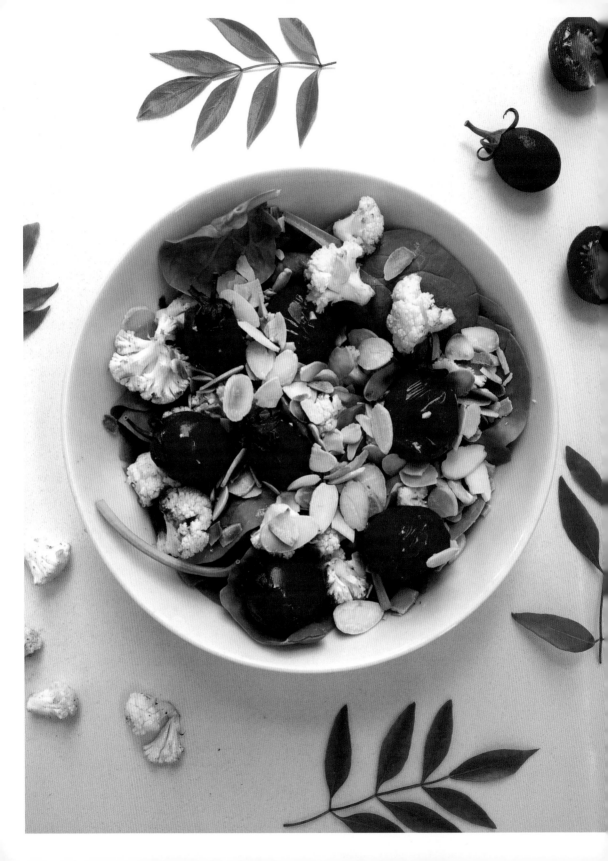

ROASTED TOMATO AND CUMIN CAULIFLOWER SALAD

INGREDIENTS

1 head of cauliflower

Large handful of baby tomatoes

2 tablespoons (30 ml) of olive oil

1 teaspoon (5 ml) of cumin powder

Salt and pepper to taste

Fresh spinach

2 tablespoons (30 ml) of flaked almonds

Avocado or animal protein of choice (optional)

METHOD

Preheat the oven to 350 degrees F (180 degrees C).

Break the cauliflower into florets and add to a baking dish alongside the tomatoes. Drizzle with olive oil and add the cumin, salt, and pepper. Roast for 10-15 minutes. Let cool when finished cooking.

In a large bowl, add your desired amount of spinach followed by the cauliflower and tomatoes and avocado or animal protein of choice. Toss the ingredients, and garnish with flaked almonds.

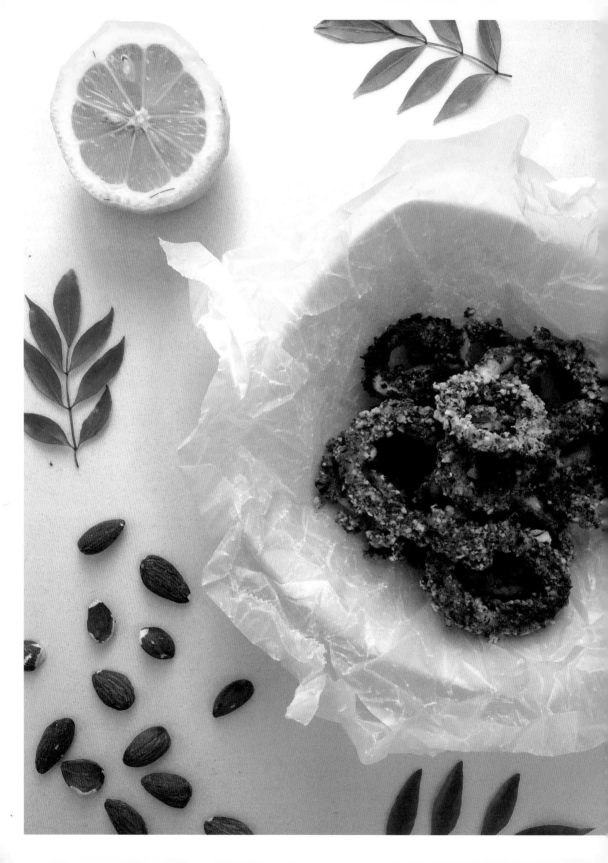

SALT AND PEPPER SQUID

SERVES 2

INGREDIENTS

1/2 cup (75 g) almonds

1 handful of fresh thyme or 2 teaspoons (10 ml) of dried herb

1 handful of fresh chives or 2 teaspoons (10 ml) of dried herb

1 teaspoon (5 ml) Himalayan salt

1 teaspoon (5 ml) black pepper

1 egg

10 ounces (300 grams) calamari rings

METHOD

Blend all the ingredients in a food processor (except the eggs and calamari) into a crumb like mixture—set aside.

Whisk the egg in a bowl and dip the calamari rings into the egg batter. Then roll the calamari rings through the crumb mixture.

Heat the olive oil or ghee in a pan and cook the "breaded" calamari rings for 1 to 2 minutes.

Enjoy with salad.

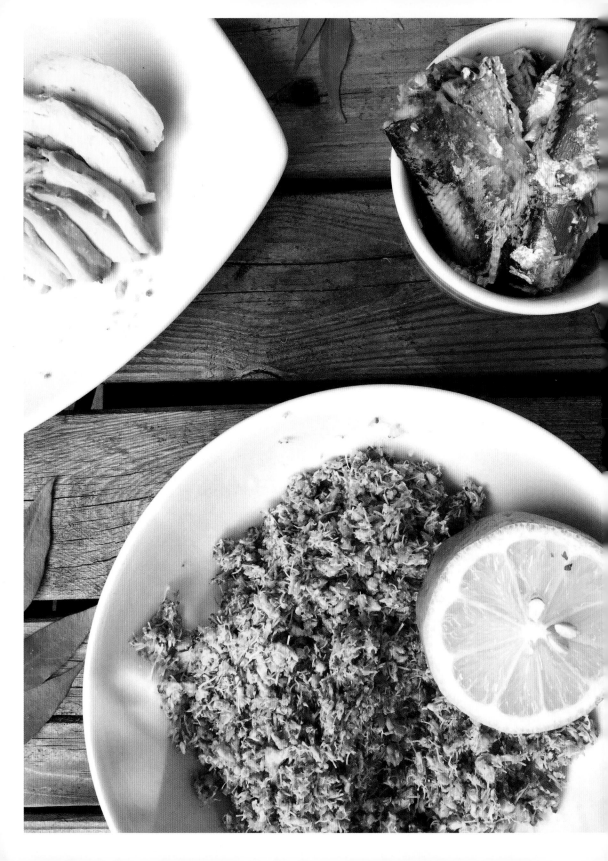

SARDINES WITH YELLOW RICE

SERVES 2

INGREDIENTS

1 medium head broccoli

1 tablespoon (15 ml) turmeric powder

Salt and pepper to taste

1 tablespoon (15 ml) coconut oil or ghee

2 cans wild sardines

1 avocado

METHOD

In a food processor, blend broccoli, turmeric, salt, and pepper into a rice-like consistency. Gently sauté the ingredients from the food processor in a pan with some ghee or coconut using a lid for a steaming effect, until soft.

Serve alongside sardines, 1 can per person, and sliced avocado for a filling, healthy-fat-filled dinner.

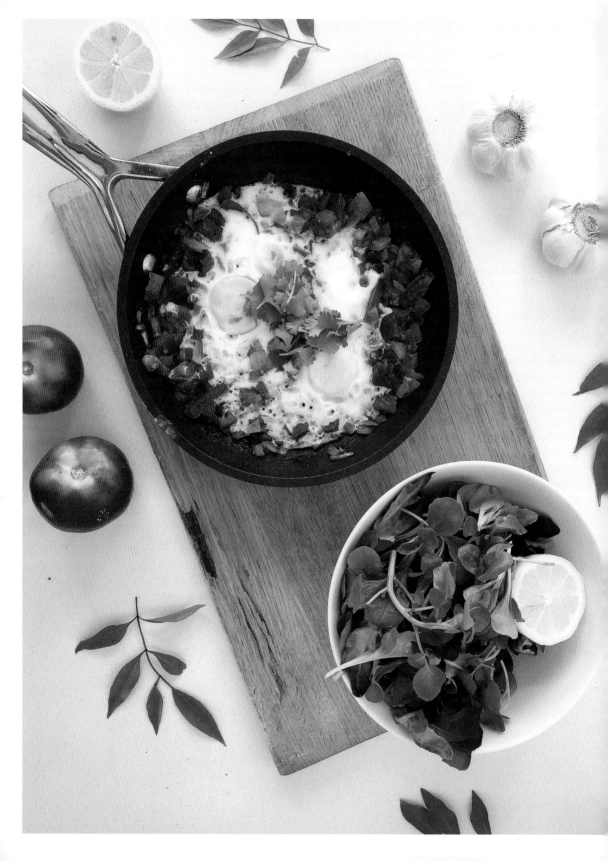

SHUKSHUKA

SERVES 2

INGREDIENTS

4 tablespoons (60 ml) of olive oil, for frying

1 small onion, chopped

3 cloves garlic, crushed and coarsely chopped

5 large tomatoes, diced thinly

1/2 teaspoon (2 ml) Himalayan salt

Pinch of:

    cayenne

    paprika

    cumin

    black pepper

6 eggs

METHOD

Heat oil in a saucepan over medium-low heat. Sauté the onions, stirring occasionally for two minutes before adding the garlic and stirring frequently for another minute or so. Now stir in the tomatoes, salt, and rest of the spices and let simmer for another five to six minutes to allow the mixture to thicken.

Create some small indents or pockets in the sauce with the back of a spoon, and then crack an egg into each indent. Place a lid on the saucepan to poach the eggs for a further 3 to 5 minutes. Serve alongside a light, easy salad.

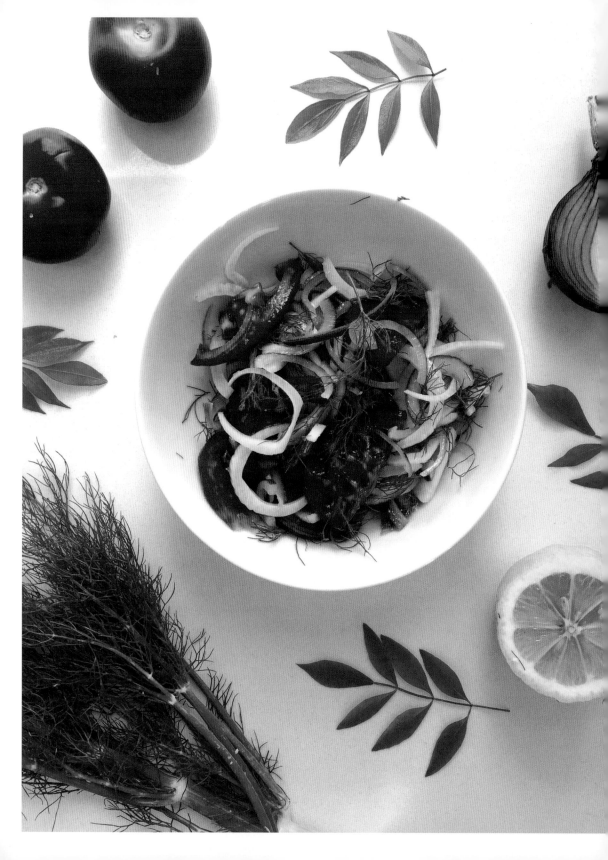

TOMATO, RED ONION, AND FENNEL SALAD

SERVES 2

INGREDIENTS

1 fennel bulb

2 large tomatoes

1/2 red onion

2 tablespoons (30 ml) of finely chopped fennel leaves

Half a lemon, juiced

1 tablespoon (15 ml) olive oil

1/2 teaspoon (2 ml) sea salt

Animal protein of your choice (optional)

METHOD

Very finely slice the fennel bulb, fennel leaves, tomatoes and red onion.

Add to a bowl and squeeze the lemon juice over, drizzle with olive oil, and add the salt.

Stir to combine, and serve with an animal protein of your choice.

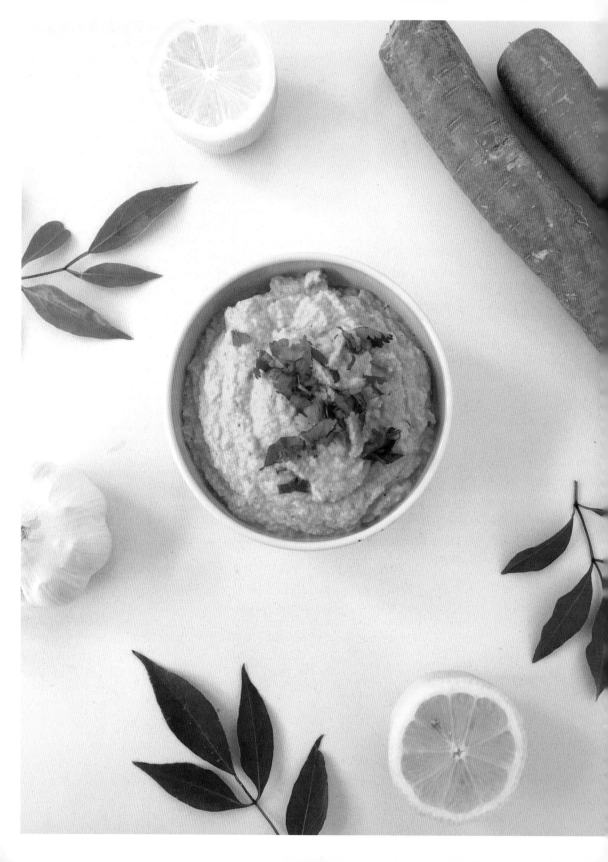

YELLOW CARROT DIP

MAKES 1 LARGE BOWL

INGREDIENTS

4 large carrots, chopped

1 whole lemon including rind, sliced

2 cloves garlic

1-inch (3 cm) piece of ginger

1-inch (3 cm) piece turmeric or 1 teaspoon turmeric powder

2 big handfuls of fresh cilantro

3/4 cup (175 ml) olive oil

METHOD

Blend together and enjoy as a salad dressing or as a dip for carrots and celery!

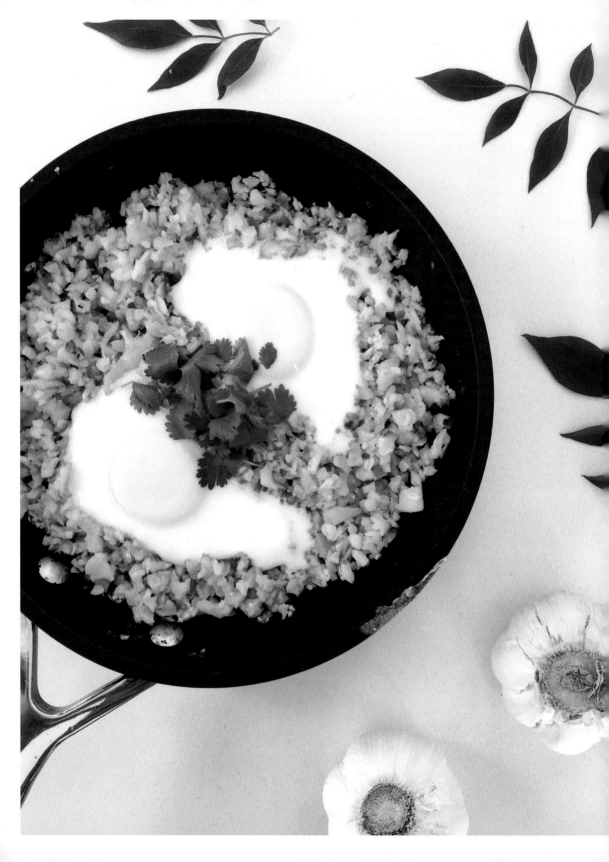

YELLOW CAULI RICE

SERVES 2

INGREDIENTS

1 medium cauliflower

2 cloves of garlic

1-inch (3 cm) piece of fresh turmeric

1 teaspoon (5 ml) turmeric powder

1 teaspoon (5 ml) Himalayan salt

1 tablespoon (15 ml) ghee or coconut oil

4 eggs

METHOD

Process all the ingredients, except the eggs, in a food processor until "rice-like."

Transfer the ingredients to a pan and sauté over medium heat for 3 to 4 minutes.

Create slight indents in the rice for your eggs, crack them in there, and cover the pan with a lid.

Let sit for 2 to 3 minutes before serving.

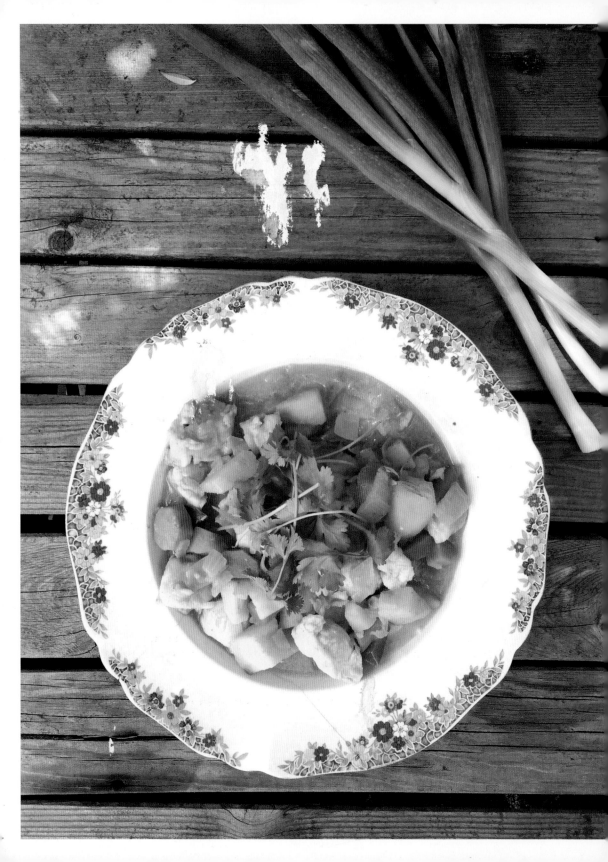

YELLOW FISH CURRY

SERVES 2

INGREDIENTS

2 tablespoons (30 ml) ghee or coconut oil

1 brown onion

1 small-medium sweet potato

1 carrot

8.5 fluid ounces (250 ml) bone broth (fish broth works best)

1 tablespoon (15 ml) turmeric powder

1 tablespoon (15 ml) curry powder

2 whole lemons

2 spring onions

7 fluid ounces (200ml) coconut cream

1 teaspoon (5 ml) Himalayan salt

1.1 pound (500 g) snapper (or white fish of choice)

1/2 bunch cilantro

Black pepper to taste

METHOD

Chop the vegetables as desired for your curry.

Heat the oil in a pot and lightly sauté the brown onion, sweet potato, and carrot for 1 to 2 minutes.

Add the bone broth, turmeric and curry powders, quartered lemon, spring onion, coconut cream, and salt, and cook for a further 10 minutes on low heat.

Chop the fish as desired and add to the pot, cooking for 1 to 2 minutes. Remove the lemons after squeezing them extra hard so that their juices flow into your curry.

Serve the curry in bowls and dress with fresh cilantro and pepper!

Sample Meal Plan—7 Days

DAY	BREAKFAST	SNACK (optional)	LUNCH	SNACK (optional)	DINNER
1	Basic Eggs	Handful of soaked nuts	Red Prebiotic Salad	1 cup Bone Broth	Coconut Lime Chicken Soup
2	Coconut Lime Chicken Soup (leftovers)	Handful Chili Nut Mix	Rainbow Salad with Almond Brazil Pesto	Flax Crackers with Yellow Carrot Dip	Yellow Fish Curry
3	Shukshuka	1 cup Bone Broth	Yellow Fish Curry (leftovers)	Kale Chips	Rainbow Salad
4	Chia Pudding	Handful of soaked nuts	Red Prebiotic Salad	1 cup Bone Broth	Lettuce Tacos
5	Green Smoothie + handful of almonds	1 cup Bone Broth	Lettuce Tacos (leftovers)	Carrot and celery sticks with Almond Brazil Pesto	Salt n Pepper Squid with Rainbow Salad
6	Basic Eggs	Handful Chili Nut Mix	Rainbow Salad with Almond Brazil Pesto	1 cup Bone Broth	Kale, Tomato, and Chicken Soup
7	Kale, Tomato, and Chicken Soup (leftovers)	Kale Chips	Rainbow Salad with sardines or tuna	Flax Crackers with Almond Brazil Pesto	Cauliflower Fritters with Red Prebiotic Salad

THE GUT HEALING PROTOCOL

CHAPTER 8

Transitioning from Gut Healing to Gut Nourishing

You may have finished what you feel is an appropriate amount of time on the Gut Healing Protocol. Your symptoms are faring much better, you generally feel more energetic and alive, and you are thinking about transitioning onto a more general gut-nourishing diet.

Although we talk about the GHP in this book as being an 8-week program, if you're like some, you'll actually need 12 to 16 weeks (sometimes longer) to fully heal. I encourage you to be honest with yourself about whether or not you're ready to finish your gut-healing journey and move into a more relaxed gut-nourishing diet.

Keep in mind, for non-athletes it takes around 120 days for your blood supply to completely renew. Your blood feeds the entire body, so it is very important in regard to overcoming illness. You may be one of those people who need to be on the GHP for the full 120 days to get the turnaround you desire.

A general rule of thumb in alternate healing circles is that for every year you've been unwell or living unhealthily, it takes one month to heal. If you've been living unhealthily for 30 years, it may well take 2-3 years for you to become well. You may not need to be on the GHP 100 percent over that time, but it certainly will help your healing journey to rebalance your microbiome.

The healthy habits that you should have learned from this protocol are fantastic for you to implement in your daily life. For instance, how much better do you feel having protein and fat for breakfast instead of carbohydrates? How much better do you feel when you follow the principle of food combining?

During your transition onto the Gut Nourishing Diet, you may wish to introduce some foods back into your regime. Sometimes, doing a good gut-healing program serves to reset the gut, and every so often this will actually highlight problem foods in the diet. Let's have a look at how you can approach the reintroduction of potentially challenging foods back into your body.

How to Identify Troublesome Foods

One of the best strategies for identifying foods that may be troublesome for you is to use Dr. Natasha Campbell-McBride's sensitivity test.[135] This involves placing a tiny amount of the food on your inner wrist before going to bed and seeing if the skin is red/irritated in the morning. You can take some egg and simply rub a tiny amount of the yolk on the skin. Although clearly, if you have extreme allergies to certain foods and are at risk for anaphylaxis, this is not advised.

If you pass this test (no irritation is detected), consume the food on an empty stomach in the morning. This is actually how I recommend consuming fruit for the most part anyway, or perhaps in a green smoothie. The reason we wouldn't be able to identify troublesome foods in a smoothie is because there are too many ingredients, and we wouldn't know which ones are causing the issue.

So, let's say you've done the GHP for 8 weeks and you're feeling ready to include some new foods back into the diet, some kiwi fruit for instance. In the morning after you have risen and drank some water, if your food sensitivity test is negative (no reaction) then you are now ready to try reintroducing that food.

Simply eat one serving of kiwi fruit and wait for 2 to 3 hours before consuming anything else. Ask yourself these questions:

How did it make me feel?

Did I feel energized?

Was my digestion sound after it…or did my belly rumble, tumble, and growl excessively at me?

How did I feel at 4 p.m. that afternoon?

Did I get an itchy throat or rash?

These are all important questions you should ask yourself, and if you have any concerns, then chances are you're not ready for that food. Remember, it is important to eat new foods on their own so that you can determine their effects on you.

You should follow this protocol for foods such as:

All fruit

Nuts

Seeds

Fermented foods (e.g., apple cider vinegar, sauerkraut, kefir)

Grains (rice, quinoa, oats)˙

If you're a health-conscious cookie, then chances are you'll probably want to indulge in a raw cake or two on occasion. I certainly do. I have to reiterate again that these foods do creep up on you and sneak back into the diet on a regular basis. Many people do genetically have a sweet tooth that has been exacerbated by years of sweet-food conditioning, so it is hard to kick; just stay in control.

This is where the idea of a "cheat day" can be beneficial for you. If you don't like the idea or name of a cheat day, then call it something else. Schedule your time "off the diet" in order to maintain a clear start and end to your indulging; this will help keep you on track for the long-term. This "time-off" can often align with a friend's wedding or birthday party, and it can help you to feel like a "normal" human.

Fermented Foods

Fermented foods, as we have spoken about throughout this book, are an awesome way for you to bring beneficial bacteria and yeast back into your body to begin widening the diversity of your microbiome. Again, we have focused more on particular strains of bacteria up until now because when someone has a leaky gut, some bacteria and yeast, although beneficial in the gut, may actually cause more harm than good if they pass through the intestinal lining into the bloodstream.

Now that we have presumably healed and sealed your gut lining, it is a great time to add these probiotic foods back into your diet as condiments to your meals.

I cover all things fermented in my book *The Art of Probiotic Nutrition: Mastering Fermented Foods for Better Digestion, Weight Control, Immunity and Longevity* which you can purchase on Amazon or from kalebrock.com. Let's go over some of the healthiest fermented foods which you should consider adding back into your diet.

Fermented Vegetables

One of the healthiest forms of fermented food is fermented or cultured vegetables. This is because you not only receive benefit from the great number of beneficial microbes growing on the vegetables, but also the pre-digested, extremely bioavailable vegetables themselves!

There are numerous ways we can create cultured vegetables, but my favorites are my kimchi and sauerkraut recipes from my book *The Art of Probiotic Nutrition*. In that book, I go into the numerous methods you can use to create fermented vegetables, so I highly recommend you check it out.

Consume fermented vegetables as a condiment to main meals. One to two tablespoons with a meal is a perfect amount to add flavor and probiotic nutrition to your plate. My personal favorite is kimchi mixed in with eggs and cauliflower rice—yum!

You can find quality cultured vegetable starters on www.kalebrock. com.au/ghp, or speak with your local health food store.

Kefir

Kefir is an ancient source of bacteria and beneficial yeast which is used as a starter to ferment milk, similar to the SCOBY found in Kombucha. The word kefir is actually derived from the Turkish word "Keyif," which means "good feeling." Some fabulous history surrounds kefir with glamorous stories of religious prophets gifting kefir to Islamic tribes in the Caucasus Mountains for strength and immunity. The revered grains were passed on from generation to generation for thousands of years before spreading throughout Asia and now eventually the world.

Kefir: Kefir is a fermented milk drink made with kefir "grains," a yeast/bacterial fermentation starter. It is prepared by inoculating cow, goat, or sheep milk with kefir grains.

Kefir is consumed widely in Russia, where the kefir "grain" or starter is used to ferment dairy milk. Kefir is unusual because it seems to blur the lines between a probiotic and a food. It is rich in microbiota but also loaded with minerals and amino acids like tryptophan! It is also rich in vitamin B12, B1, K, folic acid and pantothenic acid. Studies on kefir from as early as 1932 have shown kefir to be antimicrobial, immune-modulating, and possibly even anti-cancerous.[136]

Kefir:

- May be a suitable replacement for fermented food for those who are sensitive to wild ferments like sauerkraut and kombucha.

- May be beneficial for managing conditions such as SIBO, Crohn's, ADHD, and behavioral disorders.

- May assist in re-establishing the methylation pathways of folate for those with MTHFR.

- Contains large amounts of Bifidobacterium, an important species of bacteria which protects against leaky gut and assists in the digestion of starches.

- May assist in re-establishing gut health after antibiotic use by suppressing pathogenic microbes like *Candida albicans.*

- May assist in healthy weight management through its powerful effects on gut inflammation and insulin sensitivity.

- Useful as a potent liver tonic.

Kefir contains a wide variety of beneficial microbes such as:

- Lactococcus microbes

- Lactobacillus microbes

- Beneficial yeasts like Saccharomyces boulardii

- Bifidobacterium

Kefir and its live microbes have been extensively studied. Research by the Turkish Microbial Society found that each strain of kefir (that they used) could protect against food-borne pathogens like Staphylococcus, Salmonella, and Listeria.[137] Lactobacillus bacteria found in kefir have been shown to be protective against the sometimes-deadly Clostridium difficile infection.[139] Kefir may also protect against cancer by reducing the spread of malignant cells and may reduce blood pressure, fight weight gain, and control the growth of yeasts like Candida.[139] [140] [141] [142]

Consume *coconut kefir* or *raw milk kefir* as a stand-alone beverage first thing in the morning or before going to bed in the evenings. Do not consume water kefir as it contains too much sugar—however you can use alternative recipes for this as shown in my recipe book, *The Art of Probiotic Nutrition*. I like to have coconut kefir upon rising as an alkalizing, detoxifying, probiotic drink! I also love my Thai Kefir Coconut Soup Recipe!

For awesome healthy kefir starters, go to www.kalebrock.com.au /ghp or speak with your local health food store.

Kombucha

Kombucha is an ancient fermented food dating back to the earliest records of time! Most point to kombucha originating in China or Japan, but there are thoughts that it could have originated in Russia. Regardless of its origins, the mere fact that this product has lasted thousands of years and is still available to us today is a testament to its power.

Kombucha: Kombucha is naturally effervescent beverage produced by fermenting tea with a culture of yeast and bacteria.

The Symbiotic Colony of Bacteria and Yeast (SCOBY) is responsible for the health-giving properties of kombucha. The bacteria and yeast feed upon sugars and, as a result, produce amino acids, vitamins, enzymes, and numerous healing nutrients for the body. Using a sweet tea as a base for the SCOBY infuses that tea's "essence" into your kombucha, emphasizing its physiological effects. Using powerful herbal teas like tulsi, chamomile, and green tea impart incredibly powerful and medicinal properties to your kombucha.

But we shouldn't use white sugar in our kombucha!

Although our SCOBY does need a fuel to live and grow, that doesn't mean that our fuel has to be refined sugar, a recent invention. Using refined sugar in your kombucha recipes will create a drink that disrupts your microbiome rather than balancing the microbes. In fact, a study at Bucharest University showed that between 19-34% of the original sugar remains in Kombucha after fermenting (this obviously depends on how long you ferment it).[143]

Remember to follow the rule of food combining by not consuming starchy carbohydrates with animal protein.

We can still make healthy kombucha though! By using natural sweeteners that contain significant amounts of nutrition as well, we create a much more healing and traditional drink. In my fermented foods recipe book, *The Art of Probiotic Nutrition*, and my Fermented Foods Mastery online course on kalebrock.com, I teach you healthier options to fuel the SCOBY!

Use fermented foods sparingly, and rotate their frequency in your diet as much as possible. One to two small servings per day a few times per week is a good place to start.

Resistant Starch Foods

Foods containing resistant starch seem to have a very positive impact on the microbiome and GI tract *when beneficial microbes are in place.* Once we have re-established your microbiome, adding in some rice, oats, lentils, chickpeas, and cashews may be a beneficial step for you as you continue your health journey.[144] Be aware that these foods may cause irritation in your unique digestive system—so just ensure they pass your inner nutritionist test. Remember, also, to follow the rule of food combining by not consuming starchy carbohydrates with animal protein.

> We have been very diligent in damaging our gut lining for so many years, we need to be equally as diligent when it comes to reversing that damage with good nutrition from food and supplements.

According to Mark Sisson in *The New Primal Blueprint*, green bananas and plantains are a great source of resistant starch. He also advocates eating potatoes and rice only after they have cooled in order to render them resistant to normal digestion and ensure they travel through the small intestine reach the colon.[145]

As you continue to build the health of your microbiome on your Gut Nourishing Diet, it may be permissible to widen the variety of starches in your meals. Just be sure to monitor and understand how your body reacts to different foods and dietary approaches, ensuring that you always *eat with your microbes in mind.*

Continued Supplementation

Moving forward, probiotic supplementation should be maintained in conjunction with regular intakes of fermented food. Using therapeutic doses of powerful strains of bacteria like those mentioned throughout this book are a great way to ensure the ongoing health of your gut. Speak with your local health food store or naturopath about certain strains for your unique body, or check out kalebrock.com for more resources.

Bovine colostrum or Aloe vera may be reduced or stopped once you believe you have overcome your leaky gut condition. For reference, I cycle on and off colostrum throughout the year to maintain the health of my intestinal lining.

On the basis of the scientific research on minerals and trace elements, it is my belief that this is an area of nutrition most people need to supplement for the rest of their lives. We give camels and other livestock salt licks to supplement them with minerals and trace elements, yet for some reason human beings have trouble with the idea that we should supplement, too. Ongoing intakes of minerals and trace elements will have a huge impact on your health and wellbeing, and it is my belief it will contribute to your longevity. The Hunza tribe who we have referenced throughout this book are renowned for their long lifespans, often aging well past 120 years. Their daily access to highly mineralized water and crops fed by mineralized water is a strong argument for adding them into your life on a daily basis.

You have to remember we have been very diligent in damaging our gut lining for so many years, we need to be equally as diligent when it comes to reversing that damage with good nutrition from food and supplements.

Sample Gut Nourishing Meal Plan—7 Days

DAY	BREAKFAST	SNACK (optional)	LUNCH	SNACK (optional)	DINNER
1	Basic Eggs	Handful of soaked nuts	Red Prebiotic Salad	Green apple	Coconut Lime Chicken Soup
2	Home-made granola* with fresh berries and almond milk	Green apple or bliss ball*	Rainbow Salad with Almond Brazil Pesto and kimchi	Kale Chips	Yellow Fish Curry
3	Shukshuka	1 cup Bone Broth	Walnut, Pear, and Arugula Salad*	Celery and carrot sticks with Almond Brazil Pesto	Rainbow Salad
4	Chia Pudding with fresh berries	1 pear	Red Prebiotic Salad	1 cup Bone Broth	Mexican Tacos
5	Green Smoothie with green apple	Handful of Chili Nut Mix	Lettuce Tacos (leftovers)	Flax Crackers with beet dip*	Salt n Pepper Squid with Rainbow Salad
6	Basic Eggs	Flax Crackers with beet dip*	Rainbow Salad with Almond Brazil Pesto and sauerkraut	Kale Chips	Kale, Tomato, and Chicken Soup
7	Coconut Kefir Yogurt* with fresh fruit and crushed almonds	Handful of soaked nuts	Rainbow Salad with sardines or tuna	1 pear, bliss ball*, or raw cake* slice	Vegetable rice stir-fry*

Recipes for items not found in this book can been found using this link: kalebrock.com.au/ghp-recipes

Habits Stick

The fundamental habits of this protocol should stick with you for life.

Deep breathing before meals, eating protein and fat for breakfast, and taking measures to heal your intestinal lining are fantastic ongoing health strategies. Once you move past the "strict" stages of this protocol, you can be a little more flexible with your diet and enjoy the benefits from eating sweeter foods like fruit.

When you have a strong, healthy microbiome, you can enjoy some natural sugars, and so will your microbes!

Just keep in mind that these foods often sneak their way into our lives much more regularly than is healthy. In a wild situation, a paleolithic situation if you will, fruit would have been a scarce commodity for the most part, depending on the season and geographical region. So, consumption of it in forms that are local, organic and fresh and seasonal, is a healthy strategy for ongoing health.

Final Words

I remember what my health was like when I was 16. I used to wake up in the morning and be ravenous for food. I would eat 2 bowls of sugar-loaded cereal and be starving by 11 A.M. My energy would drop significantly by the afternoon, and I would be forced to load up on sugar for energy again. My surfs would be cut short because I would run out of energy to paddle; I'd have to come in and run to the bakery to eat. My immune system was literally shot. I had chest infections for months at a time, and my digestive system was in ruins. I was the chubby kid— or at least I had extra weight that I just couldn't burn off no matter how much I rode, ran, paddled, or swam.

Now things are very different. I can stay lean easily, and my energy levels have been through the roof for the majority of my life. My digestion is great, and my immune system is functioning again. For the most part, food is just fuel for me to achieve all the things I want to achieve in life. I've lost most of my emotional attachment to it (okay, chocolate still gets me every now and then) and can easily go without any food for half a day on a regular basis and still feel fully energized.

Not only that, but my emotions are so much more balanced now. I feel calm, collected, and able to make clear decisions every day, and this has had a flow-on effect to the people around me.

That is really what this protocol is about—allowing people to reach their full potential by changing the health of the world. Educating individuals to the point where they can go on and educate others is how we will change the world. Individuals can only create so much change, whereas communities can change the world.

> That is really what this protocol is about—allowing people to reach their full potential by changing the health of the world.

I used to teach a functional fitness class in my home town at 6:15 A.M. on Tuesdays and Thursdays. I loved it. Fitness is something that will always be close to my heart. One of our favorite exercises was to sprint while towing an old heavy boxing bag behind us along the grass. The extra weight makes you feel as if you're running uphill, and after 50 meters or so you're exhausted! Legs heavy, chest heaving, big grimace and all. If you're trying to run the race that is life and you have an imbalanced microbiome, then you are figuratively pulling that boxing bag along with you. All your efforts to attain optimal health and wellness, to have a joyful, fulfilling life are hindered when you're dragging that extra weight. I cannot emphasize enough that balancing the microbiome and healing the gut will assist you in creating the life that you want.

In the health world now there is certainly a growing movement of like-minded individuals sharing a similar health and wellness message, however unfortunately we also have the good old egos involved in these communities. Rather than all of us joining together under the common banner of helping people attain wellness, we're bickering and arguing over insignificant details surrounding diet, exercise, and emotions. But instead if we can achieve the singular goal of encouraging every single person in the world to at least make conscious decisions regarding their food, then we've done a good thing and have made huge strides in the right direction. Just because someone doesn't eat exactly like you, or doesn't live by the same philosophies or religion, it doesn't mean they deserve our judgement. In fact, when we give weight and energy to a judgmental thought we only exacerbate the problem. It is my belief that as soon as we begin to accept each other for who and where we are, then we will achieve a happy, healthy, and peaceful world.

Currently, we have a sick, tired, and ailing population, yet we can change this within a generation. It doesn't matter if you think lamb is better than chicken, or if you think tofu is better than egg, *if people can become informed about the food they eat* and how it affects their body outcomes, then they *will* improve their health.

The Gut Healing Protocol is everything that I've learned about health and wellness as a journalist and health coach put into a simple book to help kickstart you on your journey, progress to higher levels of health, and maintain health and wellness for the rest of your life. My job is to simply point you in the right direction, and encourage you to take charge of your health as you power into the future; I hope I've been able to do that with this book.

You deserve to be healthy, happy, and fully energized every single day.

Resources

Gut Healing Protocol Resource Page
Resources for the GHP, including links to supplements, health products, and further reading can be found at www.kalebrock.com.au/ghp.

Gut Healing Protocol Online Program
With online video lectures, shopping lists, and recipe guides, the online GHP is the perfect tool to help you on your gut-healing journey! Check it out at kalebrock.com.

Fermented Food ECourse and *The Art of Probiotic Nutrition* Book
Ready to take your gut health to the next level with fermented foods? Take the E-Course! Full of awesome fermented food recipes, demonstrated visually for you in the kitchen, plus info pages, a social media support group, and more. It'll make your transition to probiotic living easy as pie! www.kalebrock.com.au/ghp

The Podcast and Social Media
Check out my regular podcast on iTunes! I interview experts on wellness, excellence, and more! www.kalebrock.com.au/the-podcast

Check out my social media pages on Instagram and Facebook @kalesbroccoli.

Hashtag #8weekghp with your food, lifestyle, and progress photos! See Taela's and Nick's photos on the next page.

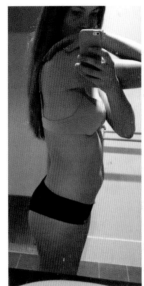
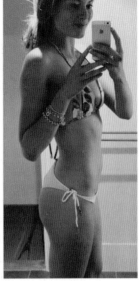

Taela

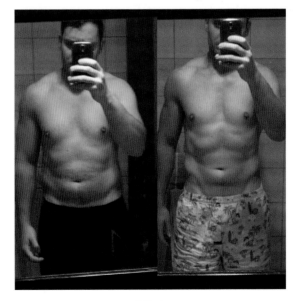

Nick

Acknowledgments

This book would not have been possible without my amazing family, friends, and colleagues.

To Eris Watkins, who taught me so much of this information and pointed me in the right direction, thank you. To Dr. Damian Kristof, thank you for being an amazing mentor.

To Ryan, Inessa, Emma, David, Dianne, Lyn, Noel, Paul, Kylie, and Zia—thank you for being there for me.

To David, Jason, Ryan, and all my friends who have contributed ideas and messages of support for this book—thank you.

To Kenya Addison, @rhythmoffood, thank you for taking the most beautiful recipe photos which I could never have taken—your work was invaluable in creating a beautiful, aesthetically appealing book.

This book would also not be possible without you, the enthusiastic reader. Thank you for taking the time to read this. I hope you've enjoyed it and found it useful and worthy of sharing.

About the Author

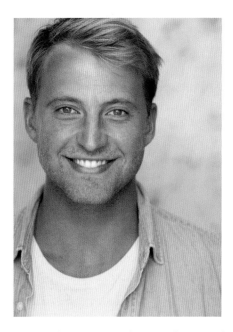

Kale Brock is an award-nominated journalist, producer, and speaker. With qualifications as a Health and Exercise coach, Kale has worked in the health and wellness industry since 2007 alongside some of the best naturopaths and health personalities in the world. Now specializing in the areas of gut health and the microbiome, Kale shares a well-rounded and comprehensive message on these areas with the general public.

Kale's books *The Gut Healing Protocol* and *The Art of Probiotic Nutrition* have generated international acclaim.

He has worked as a producer, TV host, public speaker, health and exercise coach, personal development strategist, and is an inspiring and entertaining speaker.

Kale's recent documentary "The Gut Movie" has generated world interest and acclaim.

See testimonials for Kale's work at kalebrock.com.au/changedlives.

Notes

[1] ABC News, (2014). *Gut organisms could be key to unlocking Western diseases.* [online] Available at: http://www.abc.net.au/news/2014-10-25/ gut-microbiota-linked-to-health-autism-schizophrenia/5841264

[2] World Health Organization, (2015). *Antimicrobial resistance.* [online] Available at: http://www.who.int/mediacentre/factsheets/fs194/en/

[3] News Center, Stanford (2010). *Scientists show how antibiotics enable pathogenic gut infections.* [online] Available at: http://med.stanford.edu/ news/all-news/2013/09/scientists-show-how-antibiotics- enable-pathogenic-gut-infections.html

[4] Use of Antibiotics and Risk of Type 2 Diabetes: A Population-Based Case-Control Study: The Journal of Clinical Endocrinology and Metabolism: Vol 100, No 10. (2015). The Journal of Clinical Endocrinology and Metabolism. [online] Available at: http://press. endocrine.org/doi/10.1210/jc.2015-2696 [Accessed 22 Dec. 2015].

[5] Arrieta, M. (2006). Alterations in intestinal permeability. Gut, 55(10), pp.1512-1520.

[6] World Health Organization, (2015). *Antimicrobial resistance.* [online] Available at: http://www.who.int/mediacentre/factsheets/fs194/en/

[7] McKenna, Maryn. "TED: What Do We Do When Antibiotics Don't Work Anymore?". 2015. Online Presentation.

[8] Blaser, M. (n.d.). Missing microbes.

[9] Abc.net.au, (2015). Catalyst – Special Edition – Gut Reaction. [online] Available at: http://www.abc.net.au/catalyst/gut_reaction_part_1/

[10] Abc.net.au, (2015). Catalyst – Special Edition – Gut Reaction. [online] Available at: http://www.abc.net.au/catalyst/gut_reaction_part_1/

[11] David Perlmutter M.D., (2015). The One Probiotic Supplement You Need to be Taking. [online] Available at: http://www.drperlmutter.com/ consider-lactobacillus-plantarum/?hvid=5qELg2

[12] *Probiotic Science w Microbiologist John Ellerman*, (2015). [Podcast program] The Kale Brock Show.

[13] Lee, Jae et al. "Neuro-Inflammation Induced By Lipopolysaccharide Causes Cognitive Impairment Through Enhancement Of Beta-Amyloid Generation." *Journal of Neuroinflammation* 5.1 (2008): 37.

[14] Neu, J. and Rushing, J. (2011). Cesarean Versus Vaginal Delivery: Long-term Infant Outcomes and the Hygiene Hypothesis. *Clinics in Perinatology*, 38(2), pp.321-331.

[15] *Probiotic Science w Microbiologist John Ellerman*, (2015). [Podcast program] The Kale Brock Show.

[16] Enders, G., Enders, J. and Shaw, D. (n.d.). *Gut*, location 1763-1767.

[17] Medical News Today, (2013). C-Section Babies At High Risk Of Obesity. [online] Available at: http://www.medicalnewstoday.com/ articles/261033.php

[18] "WHO Statement On Caesarean Section Rates." *World Health Organization*. N.p., 2016

[19] Ibid.

[20] Mueller, N., Bakacs, E., Combellick, J., Grigoryan, Z. and Dominguez-Bello, M. (2015). The infant microbiome development: mom matters. Trends in Molecular Medicine, 21(2), pp.109-117.

[21] Enders, G., Enders, J. and Shaw, D. (n.d.). *Gut*, location 1855-1855.

[22] Stojanović, N., Plećaš, D. and Plešinac, S. (2012). Normal vaginal flora, disorders and application of probiotics in pregnancy. Arch Gynecol Obstet, 286(2), pp.325-332.

[23] Abrahamsson, T., Jakobsson, T., Böttcher, M., Fredrikson, M., Jenmalm, M., Björkstén, B. and Oldaeus, G. (2007). Probiotics in prevention of IgE-associated eczema: A double-blind, randomized, placebo-controlled trial. Journal of Allergy and Clinical Immunology, 119(5), pp.1174-1180.

[24] Mercola.com, (2015). *Dr. Natasha Campbell-McBride on GAPS Nutritional Program*. [online] Available at: http://articles.mercola.com/sites/articles/archive/2011/07/31/dr-natasha-campbell-mcbride-on-gaps-nutritional-program.aspx

[25] Ibid.

[26] Is the gut microbiome key to modulating vaccine efficacy? (2015). *Expert Review of Vaccines*. [online] Available at: http://www.tandfonline.com/doi/full/10.1586/14760584.2015.1040395

[27] Humphries, S. and Bystrianyk, R. (n.d.). *Dissolving illusions*.

[28] NPR.org, (2014). *Modern Medicine May Not Be Doing Your Microbiome Any Favors*. [online] Available at: http://www.npr.org/2014/04/14/302899093/modern-medicine-may-not-be-doing-your-microbiome-any-favors

[29] Mercola.com, (2015). *Dr. Natasha Campbell-McBride on GAPS Nutritional Program*. [online] Available at: http://articles.mercola.com/sites/articles/archive/2011/07/31/dr-natasha-campbell-mcbride-on-gaps-nutritional-program.aspx

[30] Humphries, S. and Bystrianyk, R. (n.d.). *Dissolving illusions*.

[31] Bought Movie – The Truth Behind Vaccines, Big Pharma and Your Food. (2015). [online] Available at: http://www.boughtmovie.com

[32] Neu, J. and Rushing, J. (2011). Cesarean Versus Vaginal Delivery: Long-term Infant Outcomes and the Hygiene Hypothesis. *Clinics in Perinatology*, 38(2), pp.321-331.

[33] Enders, G., Enders, J. and Shaw, D. (n.d.). *Gut*, location 599-600.

[34] Gordon, J. (2013). Gut Microbiota from Twins Discordant for Obesity Modulate Metabolism in Mice. Science, 341(6150).

[35] Enders, G., Enders, J. and Shaw, D. (n.d.). *Gut*, location 1796-1798.

[36] Ibid.

[37] Spector, T. (n.d.). *The diet myth*, location 1670-1674.

[38] Barford, E. (2013). Parasite makes mice lose fear of cats permanently. Nature.

[39] http://www.apa.org, (2015). That gut feeling. [online] Available at: http://www.apa.org/monitor/2012/09/gut-feeling.aspx

[40] Perlmutter, D. and Loberg, K. (n.d.). *Grain brain.*

[41] Lee, Jae et al. "Neuro-Inflammation Induced By Lipopolysaccharide Causes Cognitive Impairment Through Enhancement Of Beta-Amyloid Generation." *Journal of Neuroinflammation* 5.1 (2008): 37.

[42] Jones, N. (2011). Friendly bacteria cheer up anxious mice. Nature.

[43] ScienceDaily. (2016). Do microbes control our mood? [online] Available at: https://www.sciencedaily.com/releases/2016/10/161020114611.htm

[44] Akbari, E., Asemi, Z., Daneshvar Kakhaki, R., Bahmani, F., Kouchaki, E., Tamtaji, O., Hamidi, G. and Salami, M. (2016). Effect of Probiotic Supplementation on Cognitive Function and Metabolic Status in Alzheimer's Disease: A Randomized, Double-Blind and Controlled Trial. Frontiers in Aging Neuroscience, 8.

[45] Abc.net.au, (2015). Catalyst – Special Edition – Gut Reaction. [online] Available at: http://www.abc.net.au/catalyst/gut_reaction_part_1/

[46] Oksaharju, A. (2016). Probiotic Lactobacillus rhamnosus downregulates FCER1 and HRH4 expression in human mast cells.

[47] Zajac, A., Adams, A. and Turner, J. (2016). A systematic review and meta-analysis of probiotics for the treatment of allergic rhinitis.

[48] "Leo Galland MD: Unlock Your Health." *Dr Galland.*

[49] "Media Release: Oral Therapy Could Provide Treatment For Peanut Allergies | Murdoch Childrens Research Institute." Mcri.edu.au.

[50] Spector, T. (n.d.). *The diet myth, l*ocation 2312-2318.

[51] http://journals.lww.com/co-clinicalnutrition/Abstract/2012/09000/Butyrate_implications_for_intestinal_function.13.aspx

[52] Enders, G., Enders, J. and Shaw, D. (n.d.). *Gut,* location 475-476.

[53] *Probiotic Science w Microbiologist John Ellerman*, (2015). [Podcast program] The Kale Brock Show.

[54] Ghannoum, M. A. "Bacteriome And Mycobiome Interactions Underscore Microbial Dysbiosis In Familial Crohn'S Disease." mBio 7.5 (2016): e01250-16.

[55] Ibid.

[56] Kellman, R. (n.d.). *The microbiome diet.*

[57] UW School of Medicine and Public Health, (2015). University of Wisconsin School of Medicine and Public Health. [online] Available at: http://www.med.wisc.edu/news-events/does-living-down-on-the-farm-lead-to-healthier-immune-systems-in-kids/40798

[58] Davis, W. (2011). *Wheat belly.* Emmaus, Penn.: Rodale.

[59] Catalyst: Gluten: A Gut Feeling, (2015). [TV program] ABC.

[60] Ibid.

[61] Ibid.

[62] Perlmutter, D. and Loberg, K. (n.d.). *Grain brain.*

[63] Kellman, R. (n.d.). *The microbiome diet.*

[64] Day, P. (2001). Health wars. Tonbridge, Kent, England: Credence Publications, p.70.

[65] Wolfe, D. (2008). The Sunfood Diet Success System. 7th ed. San Diego: Sunfood Publishing, p.325.

[66] Oregonstate.edu, (2015). Fat, sugar cause bacterial changes that may relate to loss of cognitive function | News and Research Communications | Oregon State University. [online] Available at: http://oregonstate.edu/ua/ncs/archives/2015/jun/fat-sugar-cause-bacterial-changes-may-relate-loss-cognitive-function

[67] Price, W. (2008). *Nutrition and physical degeneration.* Lemon Grove, CA: Price-Pottenger Nutrition Foundation.

[68] Simoncini, T. (2015). candida – Dr Simoncini Sodium Bicarbonate Cancer Therapy. [online] Curenaturalicancro.com. Available at: http://www.curenaturalicancro.com/en/candida-albicans-microbiological/

[69] "Green Tea EGCG, T Cells, And T Cell-Mediated Autoimmune Diseases. – Pubmed – NCBI." Ncbi.nlm.nih.gov. N.p., 2016.

[70] Enders, G., Enders, J. and Shaw, D. (n.d.). *Gut.*

[71] Mercola, J. (2016). Artificial Sweeteners -- More Dangerous than You Ever Imagined. [online] Mercola.com. Available at: http://articles.mercola.com/sites/articles/archive/2009/10/13/artificial-sweeteners-more-dangerous-than-you-ever-imagined.aspx

[72] Suez J, S. (2016). Artificial sweeteners induce glucose intolerance by altering the gut microbiota. – PubMed – NCBI. [online] Ncbi.nlm.nih.gov. Available at: http://www.ncbi.nlm.nih.gov/pubmed/

[73] Douard, V. and Ferraris, R. (2008). Regulation of the fructose transporter GLUT5 in health and disease. *AJP: Endocrinology and Metabolism*, 295(2), pp.E227-E237.

[74] CSIRO, "The Hungry Microbiome." N.p., 2016. Online www.csiro.au/hungrymicrobiome

[75] Spector, T. (n.d.). *The diet myth.*

[76] O'Young, R. (2015). pH Miracle: Alkaline Health, Diet, and Nutritional Supplements like greens drink and water ionizers for weight loss, diabetes, cancer, and improved health. [online] Phmiracleliving.com. Available at: http://www.phmiracleliving.com

[77] Simoncini, T. (2015). candida – Dr Simoncini Sodium Bicarbonate Cancer Therapy. [online] Curenaturalicancro.com. Available at: http://www.curenaturalicancro.com/en/candida-albicans-microbiological/

[78] EurekAlert!, (2015). Biologists ID defense mechanism of leading fungal pathogen. [online] Available at: http://www.eurekalert.org/pub_releases/2004-06/ru-bid062504.php

[79] Affairs, H. (2015). Genetic Secrets of Killer Fungus Found. [online] News. harvard.edu. Available at: http://news.harvard.edu/gazette/1997/10.30/GeneticSecretso.html

[80] Gates, D. (2006). The Largely Unknown Health Epidemic Affecting Almost ALL Americans. [online] All Body Ecology Articles. Available at: http://bodyecology.com/articles/unknown_health_epidemic.php

[81] Mendick, R. (2015). *Cooking with vegetable oils releases toxic cancer-causing chemicals, say experts.* [online] Telegraph.co.uk. Available at: http://www.telegraph.co.uk/news/health/news/11981884/Cooking-with-vegetable-oils-releases-toxic-cancer-causing-chemicals-say-experts.html

[82] Spector, T. (n.d.). *The diet myth,* location 1441-1450.

[83] Journals.cambridge.org, (2015). Vitamins A, E and fatty acid composition of the eggs of caged hens and pastured hens. [online] Available at: http://journals.cambridge.org/action/displayAbstract?fromPage=online&aid=7219036

[84] Perlmutter, D. (2015). *Keep Yourself in Ketosis.* [online] David Perlmutter M.D. Available at: http://www.drperlmutter.com/keep-ketosis/

[85] Moore, J. and Westman, E. (n.d.). *Keto clarity.*

[86] Dom D'agostino on Fasting, Ketosis and The End of Cancer, (2015). [TV program] iTunes: The Tim Ferriss Show.

[87] Fat Adaptation and Sports Nutrition with Steph Lowe, (2015). [TV program] iTunes: The Kale Brock Show.

[88] Mercola.com, (2015). *Making Bone Broth May Be the Key to Improving Your Health.* [online] Available at: http://articles.mercola.com/sites/articles/archive/2014/09/21/hilary-boynton-mary-brackett-gaps-cookbook-interview.aspx

[89] Batmangheligh, F. (1992). Your Body's Many Cries For Water. Clean Earth Books.

[90] Batmanghelidj, F. and Day, P. (2008). *The essential guide to water and salt.* Tonbridge: Credence Publications.

[91] Vitalis, D. (2015). Find A Spring. [online] Findaspring.com. Available at: http://www.findaspring.com

[92] Cuervo, A., Hevia, A., López, P., Suárez, A., Diaz, C., Sánchez, B., Margolles, A. and González, S. (2015). Phenolic compounds from red wine and coffee are associated with specific intestinal microorganisms in allergic subjects. *Food Funct.*.

[93] Perlmutter, D. (2015). Coffee? Pour a Cup!. [online] David Perlmutter M.D. Available at: http://www.drperlmutter.com/coffee-pour-cup/

[94] Science News, (2015). *A Gut Feeling about Coffee.* [online] Available at: https://www.sciencenews.org/blog/food-thought/gut-feeling-about-coffee

[95] Eskelinen MH, e. (2015). Midlife coffee and tea drinking and the risk of late-life dementia: a population-based CAIDE study. – PubMed – NCBI. [online] Ncbi.nlm.nih.gov. Available at: http://www.ncbi.nlm.nih.gov/pubmed/19158424

[96] Hal Huggins, MS. "Root Canal Dangers – Weston A Price." Weston A Price. N.p., 2010. Online.

[97] Asokan S, e. (2015). Effect of oil pulling on plaque induced gingivitis: a randomized, controlled, triple-blind study. – PubMed – NCBI. [online] Ncbi.nlm.nih.gov. Available at: http://www.ncbi.nlm.nih.gov/pubmed/19336860

[98] Asokan S, e. (2015). Effect of oil pulling on halitosis and microorganisms causing halitosis: a randomized controlled pilot trial. – PubMed – NCBI. [online] Ncbi.nlm.nih.gov. Available at: http://www.ncbi.nlm.nih.gov/pubmed/21911944

[99] Marcela, J. (2015). Toxic Teeth: How a Root Canal Could Be Making You Sick. [online] Mercola.com. Available at: http://articles.mercola.com/sites/articles/archive/2015/05/31/root-canal-teeth.aspx

[100] Lipton, B. (2005). The biology of belief. Santa Rosa, CA: Mountain of Love/Elite Books.

[101] Chek, P. (2004). *How to eat, move and be healthy!*. San Diego, CA: C.H.E.K. Institute.

[102] Healthysleep.med.harvard.edu, (2015). *Why Do We Sleep, Anyway? | Healthy Sleep*. [online] Available at: http://healthysleep.med.harvard. edu/healthy/matters/benefits-of-sleep/why-do-we-sleep

[103] Chek, P. (2004). *How to eat, move and be healthy!*. San Diego, CA: C.H.E.K. Institute.

[104] Vitamin D Myths, Facts and Science with Dr John Cannell, (2015). [TV program] iTunes: The Kale Brock Show.

[105] BLAKESLEE, S. (2015). Study Offers Surprise on Working of Body's Clock. [online] Nytimes.com. Available at: http://www.nytimes. com/1998/01/16/us/study-offers-surprise-on-working-of-body-s -clock.html

[106] Vitamin D Myths, Facts and Science with Dr John Cannell, (2015). [TV program] iTunes: The Kale Brock Show.

[107] Spector, T. (n.d.). *The diet myth*, location 657-659.

[108] Ibid.

[109] Ibid.

[110] EWG, (2015). *Body Burden: The Pollution in Newborns*. [online] Available at: http://www.ewg.org/research/body-burden-pollution-newborns

[111] Frith, M. (2016). Our tests show supermarket apples are up to 10 months old – National. Sydney Morning Herald Smh.com.au. Available at: http://www.smh.com.au/news/national/supermarket-apples-10-months-old/2008/01/19/1200620272669.html

[112] *Probiotic Science w Microbiologist John Ellerman*, (2015). [Podcast program] The Kale Brock Show.

[113] Enders, G., Enders, J. and Shaw, D. (n.d.). *Gut*.

[114] Savignac, H., Corona, G., Mills, H., Chen, L., Spencer, J., Tzortzis, G. and Burnet, P. (2013). Prebiotic feeding elevates central brain derived neurotrophic factor, N-methyl-d-aspartate receptor subunit's and d-serine. Neurochemistry International, 63(8), pp.756-764.

[115] ML, A. (2015). *Effect of lactobacilli on paracellular permeability in the gut. – PubMed – NCBI.* [online] Ncbi.nlm.nih.gov. Available at: http://www.ncbi.nlm.nih.gov/pubmed/22254077

[116] David Perlmutter M.D., (2015). *The One Probiotic Supplement You Need to be Taking.* [online] Available at: http://www.drperlmutter.com/consider-lactobacillus-plantarum/?hvid=5qELg2

[117] *Probiotic Science w Microbiologist John Ellerman,* (2015). [Podcast program] The Kale Brock Show.

[118] Perlmutter, D. (2015). The 5 Best Species Of Probiotics – Dr. David Perlmutter. [online] David Perlmutter M.D. Available at: http://www.drperlmutter.com/learn/resources/probiotics-five-core-species/

[119] Kleinsmith, A. and Fox, A. (n.d.). Scientific and Medical Research Related to Bovine Colostrum. 1st ed. self.

[120] Ibid.

[121] Chapter 3 Lactose content of milk and milk products. (1988). *The American Journal of Clinical Nutrition,* [online] 48(4), pp.1099-1104. Available at: http://ajcn.nutrition.org/content/48/4/1099

[122] New Perspective in Dietary Supplementation: Bovine Colostrum and Noni Juice Synergic Protective Effects on Intestinal Epithelium and Microbiota. (2014). *Inflammation and Cell Signaling.*

[123] Bodammer, P., Maletzki, C., Kerkhoff, C. and Lamprecht, G. (2013). Sa1760 Influence of Bovine Colostrum on Tight Junction Protein Expression, Barrier Function and Intestinal Cytokine Milieu. Gastroenterology, 144(5), p.S-300.

[124] Kleinsmith, A. and Fox, A. (n.d.). Scientific and Medical Research Related to Bovine Colostrum. 1st ed. self.

[125] Gullón B, e. (2015). In vitro assessment of the prebiotic potential of Aloe vera mucilage and its impact on the human microbiota. – PubMed – NCBI. [online] Ncbi.nlm.nih.gov. Available at: http://www.ncbi.nlm.nih.gov/pubmed/25504136

[126] Adams, M. (n.d.). The Aloe Vera Miracle. 1st ed. Natural News.

[127] Muller, M. (2005). *Colloidal Minerals And Trace Elements*. Healing Arts Press.

[128] Ibid.

[129] Isaacs, T. (2015). Our Disappearing Minerals and Their Vital Health Role (Part 1). [online] NaturalNews. Available at: http://www.naturalnews.com/023237_minerals_health_soil.html

[130] Art-bin.com, (2015). *Modern Miracle Men*. [online] Available at: http://art-bin.com/art/obeach_soils.html#hit

[131] Muller, M. (2005). Colloidal Minerals And Trace Elements. Healing Arts Press, pp.1, 48-50.

[132] Ibid.

[133] Douard, V. and Ferraris, R. (2008). Regulation of the fructose transporter GLUT5 in health and disease. *AJP: Endocrinology and Metabolism*, 295(2), pp.E227-E237.

[134] Ruscio, M, MD. (2016). 1056: Dr. Michael Ruscio Previews His London Event On The Gut Microbiome, *Jimmy Moore's Livin La Vida Low Carb Show*, iTunes.

[135] Campbell-McBride, Natasha. Gut And Psychology Syndrome. [Cambridge, U.K.: Medinform Pub.], 2010. Print.

[136] Farnworth, E. (n.d.). *Scientific research on Kefir*. 1st ed. [ebook] Food Science central. Available at: http://nutrition-healing.com/scientific%20research%20on%20kefir.pdf

[137] Ulusoy, B. H., Çolak, H., Hampikyan, H., and Erkan, M. E. (2007). An in vitro study on the antibacterial effect of kefir against some food-borne pathogens. *Türk Mikrobiyoloji Cemiyeti Dergisi*, 37, 103-107.

138 Carasi, P., Trejo, F. M., Pérez, P. F., De Antoni, G. L., and Serradell, M. D. L. A. (2012). Surface proteins from *Lactobacillus kefir* antagonize *in vitro* cytotoxic effect of *Clostridium difficile* toxins. *Anaerobe, 18*(1), 135-142.

139 Maalouf, K., Baydoun, E., and Rizk, S. (2011). Kefir induces cell-cycle arrest and apoptosis in HTLV-1-negative malignant T-lymphocytes. *Cancer management and research, 3,* 39.

140 Kurtzman, C., Fell, J. W., and Boekhout, T. (Eds.). (2011). *The yeasts: a taxonomic study* (Vol. 1).

141 García-Tejedor, A., Sánchez-Rivera, L., Castelló-Ruiz, M., Recio, I., Salom, J. B., and Manzanares, P. (2014). Novel antihypertensive lactoferrin-derived peptides produced by Kluyveromyces marxianus: gastrointestinal stability profile and in vivo angiotensin I-converting enzyme (ACE) inhibition. *Journal of Agricultural and Food Chemistry.*

142 Albuquerque, P., and Casadevall, A. (2012). Quorum sensing in fungi-a review. *Medical Mycology, 50*(4), 337-345.

143 Gates, D. (2014). 4 Surprising Reasons to Ditch Kombucha. [online] All Body Ecology Articles. Available at: http://bodyecology.com/articles/4-surprising-reasons-to-ditch-kombucha

144 CSIRO, "The Hungry Microbiome." Csiro.au. N.p. Available at: http://www.csiro.au/hungrymicrobiome/index.html

145 Sisson, Mark (2017). The New Primal Blueprint. Oxnard, CA. Primal Blueprint Publishing.

Index

erythritol, 64, 69
exercise, 103–105
    BEEMS time, 105–107

F

FAQ
    babies/young children
      on GHP, 128, 129
    bloating, 127
    constipation, 122–123
    doctor recommenda-
      tions against GHP,
      127–128
    falling off/getting back
      on GHP, 125
    FODMAP diet,
      121–122
    fruit, 128
    glutamine, 121
    hunger, 127
    prebiotics vs probiotics,
      121
    pregnant on GHP, 128
    SIBO (Small Intesti-
      nal Bacterial Over-
      growth), 124
    sugar cravings, 126
    vegans, 126–127
    weight loss, 124–125
    worsening symptoms
      and Herxheimer
      reaction, 123
Fasano, Alessio, 54
fats, healthy, 73, 83
fecal matter transplants
  (FMTs), 24
feeding, 52–53
fennel
    Fennel Fish Fritters,
      155
    Tomato, Red Onion,
      and Fennel Salad, 197
fermented foods, 48–49

e-course, 219
identifying troublesome
    foods, 207
kefir, 209,–210
kombucha, 211–212
not allowed foods, 70
transitioning to Gut
    Nourishing Diet,
    208–212
vegetables, 208–209
fiber, 73–74
    smoothies, 94–95
fish, 81
    Fennel Fish Fritters,
      155
    Fish Soup, 157
    raw, 81
    Sardines with Yellow
      Rice, 193
flax seeds, 69
    Flax Crackers, 159
fluoride, 93
FODMAPs (Fermentable
  Oligosaccharides,
  Disaccharides, Monosac-
  charides, And Polyols),
  65–66, 121–122
    FODMAP-Friendly
      Red Beef Soup, 161
food allergies, 42–43
food combining, 84–85
    resistant starch foods,
      213
food lists, 68–70
Fox, Alfred, 114
fruit, 60–62, 128
    alkalinity of citrus, 76
    identifying troublesome
      foods, 207
    paleolithic situation,
      217
functional medicine, 52
fungus
    antifungal herbs, 90–92

Candida. *See* Candida
  mushrooms, 80–81

G

GABA (Gamma Amino
  Butyric Acid), 38–39, 104
Gameau, Damon, 60
GAPS (Gut and Psychol-
  ogy Syndrome) diet, 31,
  123–124
Gates, Donna, 77
gelatin, 89
ghee, 58, 69, 83
    cooking, 82
GHP (Gut Healing Proto-
  col), 1–7
    8-week GHP at a
      glance, 71
    dietary principles, 72
    doctor recommenda-
      tions against, 127–128
    fundamental principles,
      51–52
    vs. Gut Nourishing
      Diet, 65–67
    NO foods, 70
    pregnant on GHP, 128
    resources, 219
    sample meal plan, 204
    starting out, 131–133
    transitioning to Gut
      Nourishing Diet, 206
    YES foods, 68–69
GLUT-5, 122
glutamine, 121
gluten, 54–56
goat's milk, 58
Grain Brain (Perlmutter),
  56
grains, 70
    identifying troublesome
      foods, 207
    wheat, 54–57

L

lactic acid, 104
Lactobacillus, 112–113
  birth canal, 36
  Lactobacillus rhamnosus
    (LGG), 42, 43
LaFave, Dr. Robert, 117
leaky gut, 18–19, 25–27
leftovers, 74
Lettuce Tacos, 173
lipopolysaccharide (LPS),
  27–28, 40
Lipton, Dr. Bruce, 98
liver detoxes, 27
LPS (lipopolysaccharide),
  27–28, 40
lymphatic system, 104–105

M

macadamia nuts, 69
macadamia oil, 69, 83
  cooking, 82
Mackay, Charles, 17
Masai, 21
  fermented milk, 57
meal plans
  Gut Healing Protocol,
    204
  Gut Nourishing Diet,
    215
meal time
  diaphragmatic breath-
    ing, 99–100
  saying grace, 86
meat
  animal protein, 81–83
  NO list, 70
  YES list, 68
Meatloaf, 175
medicinal herbs, 90–92
metabolites, 22–23
Mexican Salsa and Guac
  with Cucumber Chips, 177

microbes
  antimicrobial resistance,
    20–21
  E. coli. *See* E. coli
  H. pylori. *See* H. pylori
  in soil, 16
  kefir, 210
  metabolites, 22–23
  probiotics. *See* probi-
    otics
  quorum sensing, 22–25
  seeding, 52
  superbugs, 20
  Zobellia, 20–21
microbiome, 3, 15–17
  4 main functions, 16
  definition, 3
  diversity, 24
  microbial influence,
    35–37
  microbiota, 3
  toxicity, 31–32
The Microbiome Diet (Kellman), 51, 55
microbiota, 3
microvilli, 45–46
milk, 57–59
minerals, 116–119
Missing Microbes (Blaser),
  22
Mixed Pepper and Basil
  Salad, 179
molecular mimicry, 25
Moore, Jimmy, 88
mothers. *See* pregnancy;
  birth/infancy
Muller, Dr. Marie-France,
  116, 118
multiple sclerosis, 62
mushrooms, 80–81
mycotoxins, 56

N

natural sugars, 217
Neu, Dr. Josef, 28, 34–35
The New Primal Blueprint
  (Sisson), 213
Nietzsche, 108
nightshades, 80–81
NO foods, 70
Northern, Dr. Charles,
  117–118
nutrient supplementation.
  See supplementation
*Nutrition and Physical
  Degeneration* (Price), 60
nuts, 69–70
  Chili Nut Mix, 149
  gut-nourishing diet vs.
    gut-healing program,
    66
  healthy fats, 83
  Homemade Almond
    Milk, 167
  identifying troublesome
    foods, 207

O

O'Young, Dr. Robert, 75
oil pulling, 96–98
oils, 69
  frying, 82
olive oil, 69, 83
  oil pulling, 96–98
omega-6/omega-3 fats,
  eggs, 86
oral biome, 96–98
organic
  bones for bone broth,
    90
  meat, 83
osteoporosis, 59

Roasted Bell Pepper, Avocado Cream, and Cilantro Salsa, 187
Roasted Tomato and Cumin Cauliflower Salad, 189
Rushing, Dr. Jona, 28, 34–35

S

saccharin, 63–64
Saccharomyces boulardii yeast, 113
salad, 74
  Mixed Pepper and Basil Salad, 179
  Rainbow Salad, 183
  Red Prebiotic Salad, 185
  Roasted Tomato and Cumin Cauliflower Salad, 189
  Tomato, Red Onion, and Fennel Salad, 197
Salmonella infections, 115
salsa
  Mexican Salsa and Guac with Cucumber Chips, 177
  Roasted Bell Pepper, Avocado Cream, and Cilantro Salsa, 187
salt
  adding to drinking water, 93, 119, 132
  mineral supplementation, 118–119
  sugar cravings, 126
Salt and Pepper Squid, 191
San, 48
Sardines with Yellow Rice, 193

SCOBY (Symbiotic Colony of Bacteria and Yeast), 211–212
seafood
  Fennel Fish Fritters, 155
  Fish Soup, 157
  raw fish, 81
  Salt and Pepper Squid, 191
  Sardines with Yellow Rice, 193
  Yellow Fish Curry, 203
seeding, 31, 52–53
seeds, 69–70
  Flax Crackers, 159
  gut-nourishing diets vs. GHP, 66
  identifying troublesome foods, 207
segmented filamentous bacteria, 28
serotonin, 38
Serratia marcescens, 46
sheep's milk, 58
Shukshuka, 195
SIBO (Small Intestinal Bacterial Overgrowth), 124
Simoncini, Dr. Tullio, 61, 77
Sisson, Mark, 213
sleep, 100–101
  sunlight, 101–102
smoothies, 94–95
  Green Smoothie, 163
soil microbes, 16
soup
  Chicken and Leek Soup, 147
  Coconut Lime Chicken Soup, 151
  Creamy Onion Soup, 153
  Fish Soup, 157

FODMAP-Friendly Red Beef Soup, 161
  Healing Kale Soup, 165
  Kale, Tomato, and Chicken Soup, 171
Spector, Dr. Tim, 75, 83, 104
spices, 69
squash, 81
squid, SALT AND PEPPER SQUID, 191
STARTING GHP, 131–133
  sample meal plan, 204
stevia, 64, 69
stomach acid, 47
storage hormone, 125
stress, 98–100
  breathing diaphragmatically, 99
  sleep, 100–101
sucralose, 63–64
sugar, 59–62
  artificial sweeteners, 63–65
  cravings, 126
  natural sugars, 217
sun exposure, 101–102
  BEEMS time, 105–107
superbugs, 20
supplementation, 109–119
  Aloe vera, 116
  bovine colostrum, 114–115
  glutamine, 121
  minerals and trace elements, 116–119
  probiotics, 111–114. *See also* probiotics
  reinoculating, 53
  replacing, 52
  transitioning to Gut Nourishing Diet, 214
sweet vegetables, 60, 62
sweeteners, 63–65